This book belongs to:

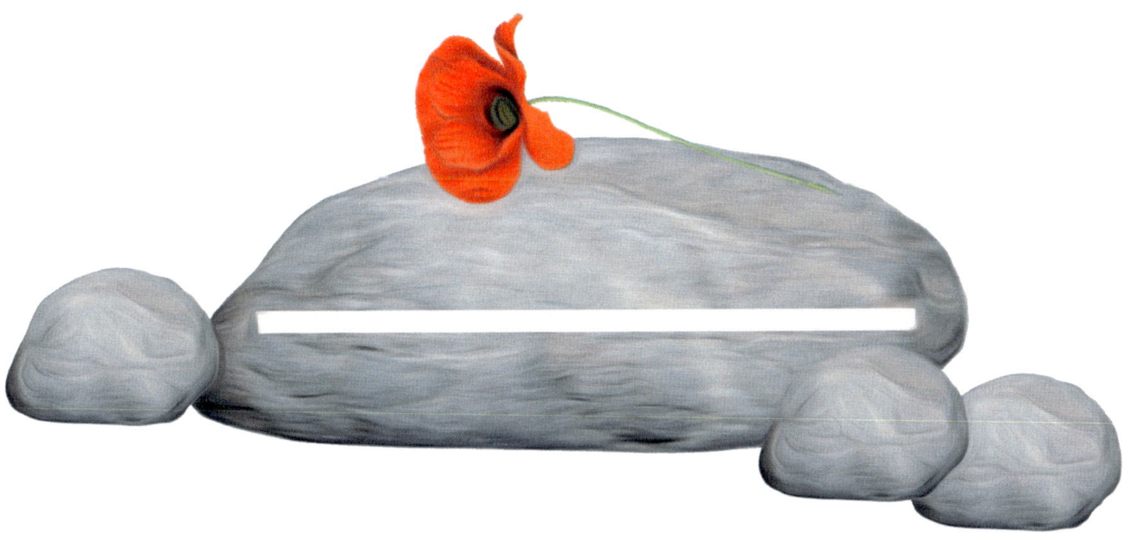

Published by AMor Rustic Arts Books - Independent Publishing Network, 2018.

Illustrated by Magdalena Adic
Writing Consultant Grace Campbell

The information in this book is the author's personal experience and thoughts. Anita Morrison (AMor Rustic Arts) is not liable or responsible for outcomes based on this book. Suitability is the responsibility of the parent/guardian.

ISBN Number: 978-1-78926-815-7

A CIP catalogue record for this book is available from the British Library.

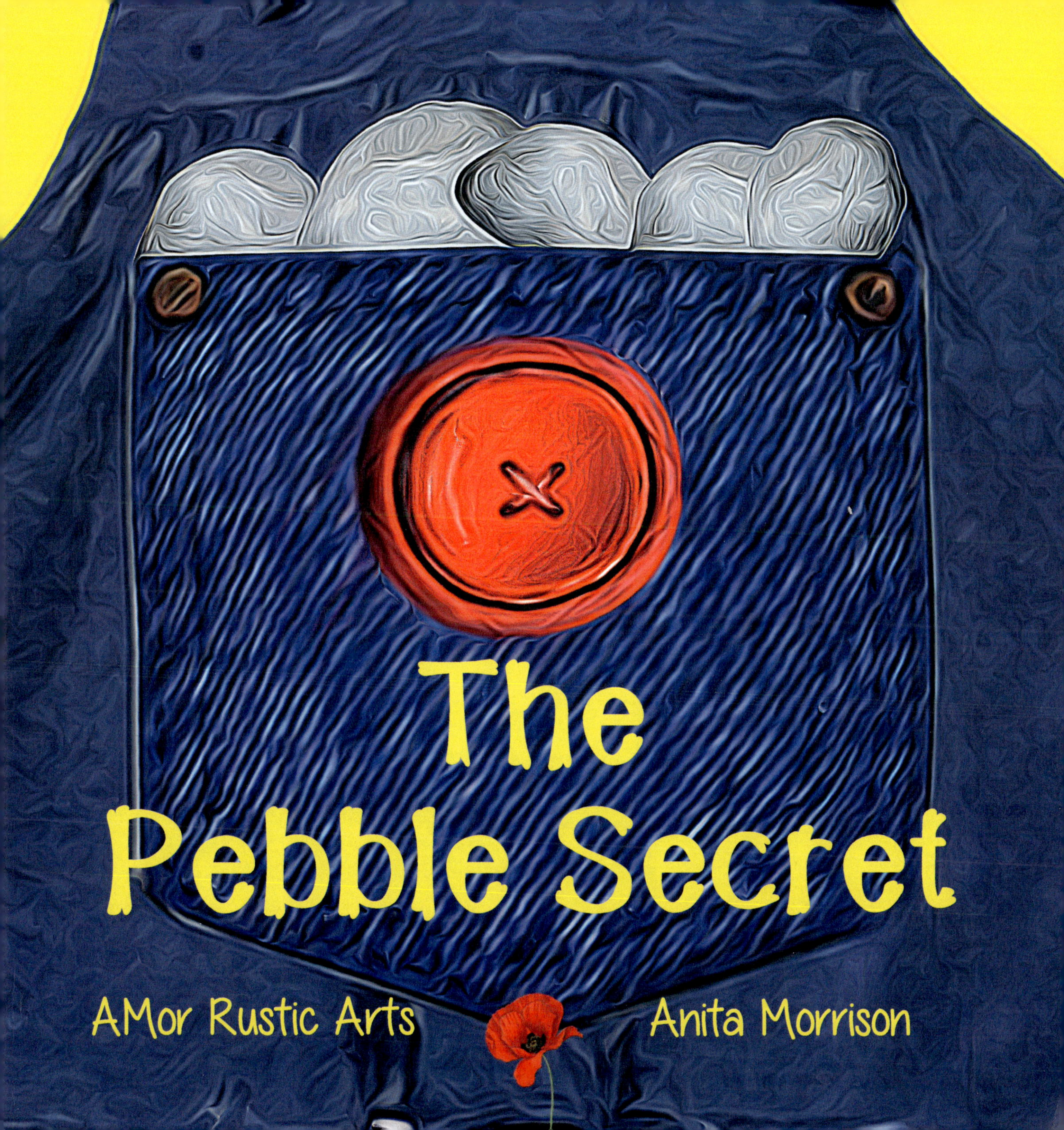
The
Pebble Secret
AMor Rustic Arts
Anita Morrison

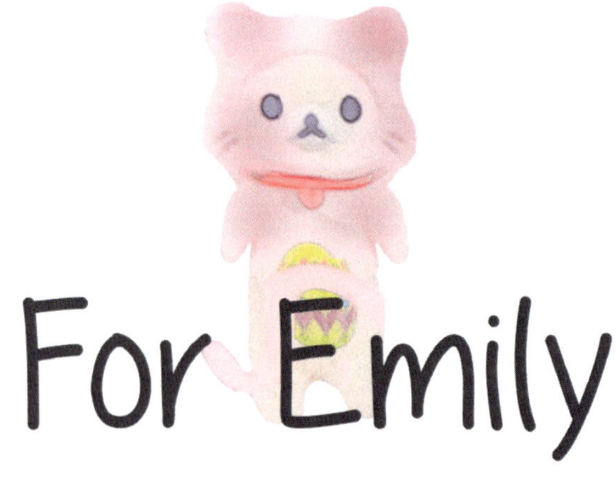

For Emily

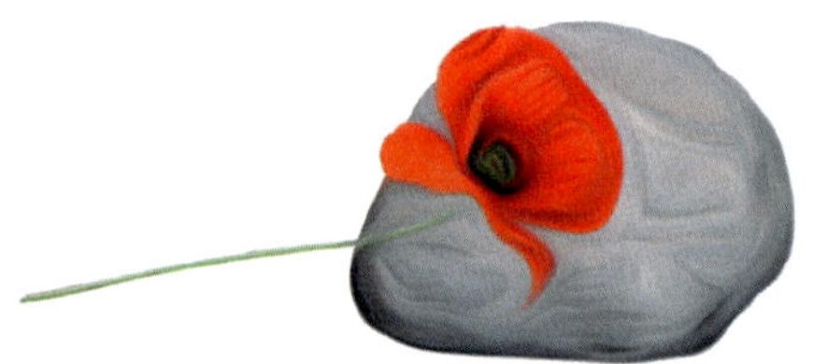

and every child who needs
to know they were
created perfectly.

There was a little girl.
She looked like any other little girl...

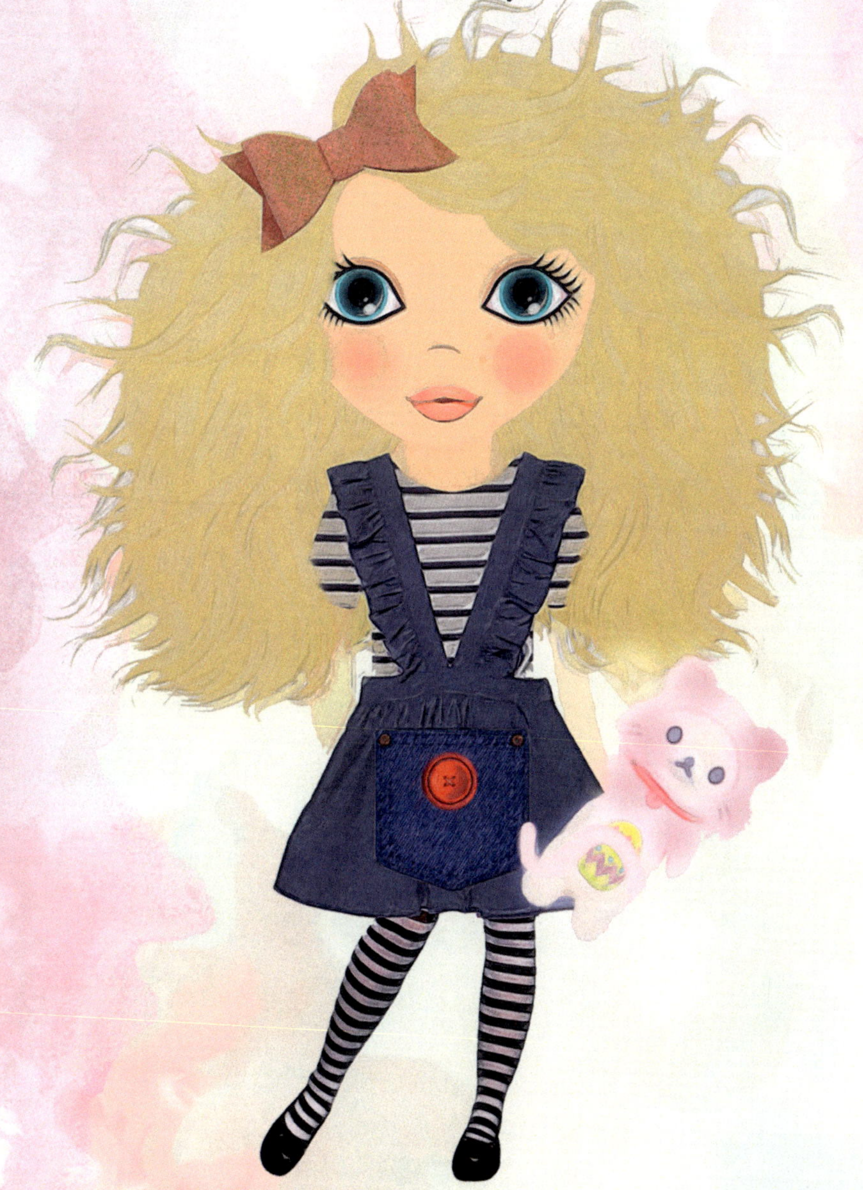

but she carried a secret not even she knew.

Not even her class at school knew.

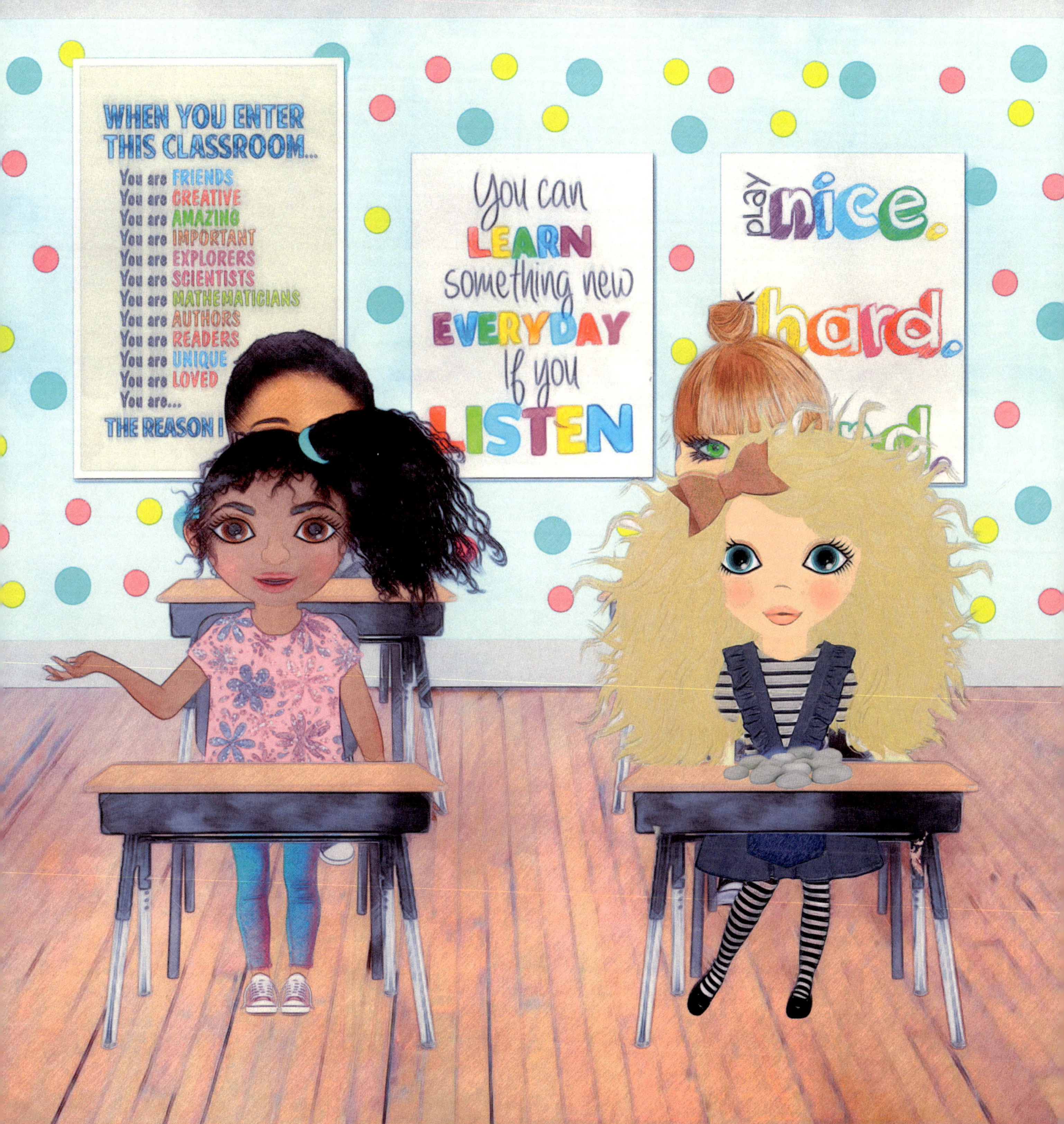
WHEN YOU ENTER THIS CLASSROOM...
You are FRIENDS
You are CREATIVE
You are AMAZING
You are IMPORTANT
You are EXPLORERS
You are SCIENTISTS
You are MATHEMATICIANS
You are AUTHORS
You are READERS
You are UNIQUE
You are LOVED
You are...
THE REASON I
You can LEARN something new EVERYDAY If you LISTEN
play nice.
hard.

She found it hard to talk to her classmates and often didn't know what to say. Her secret sometimes meant she would say silly things she thought were hilarious like...

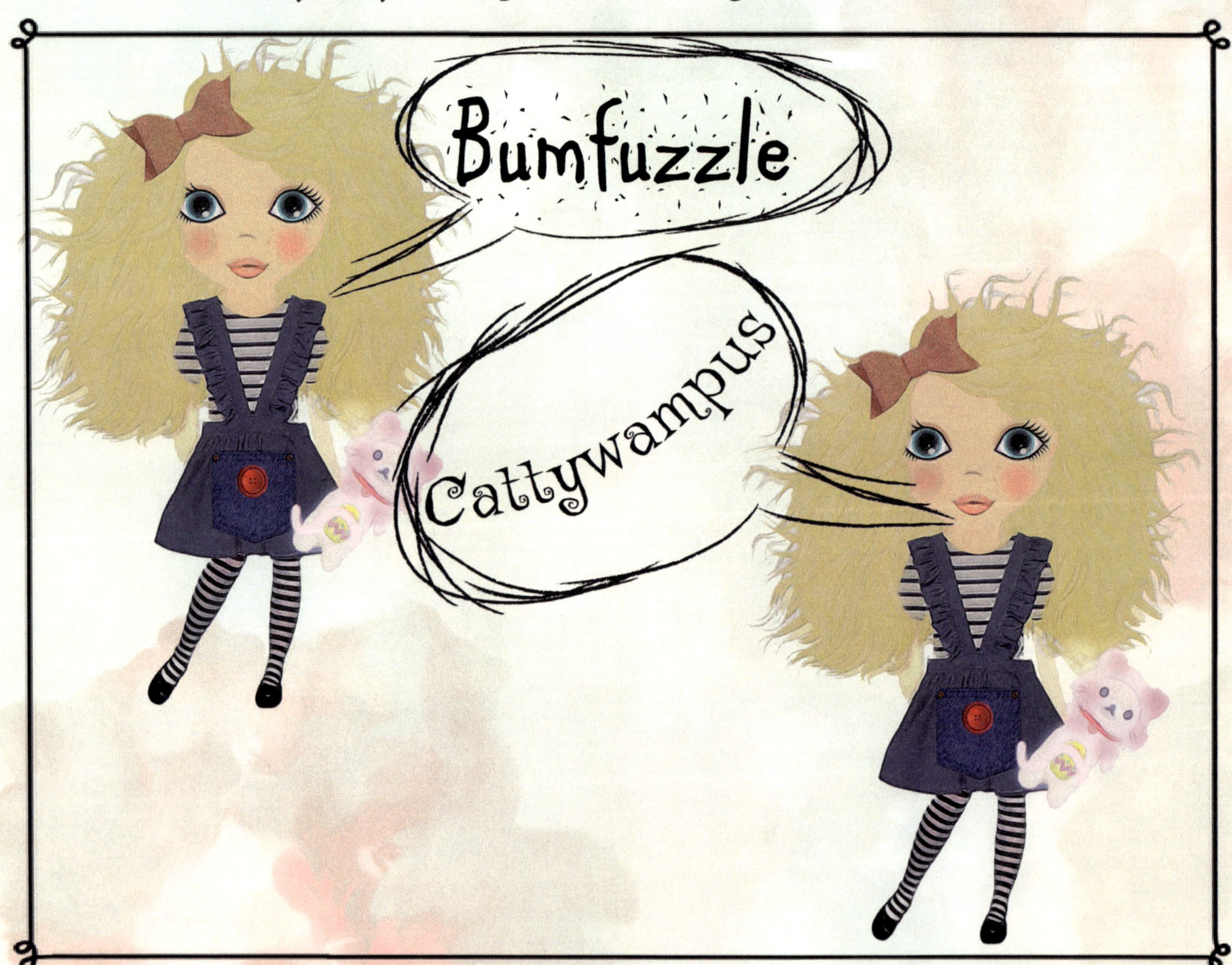

and "Imagine a dog with a pancake on its head."

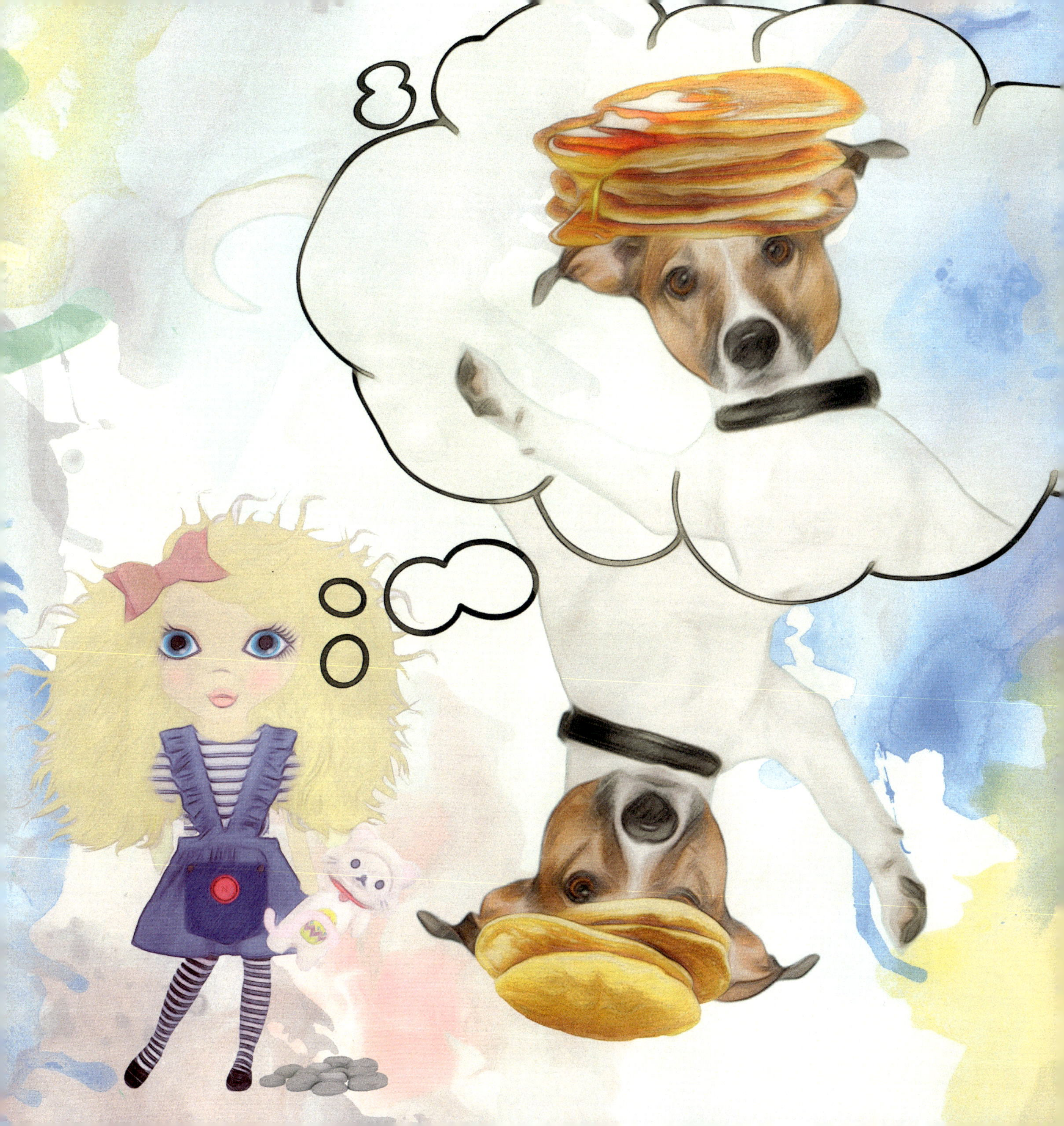

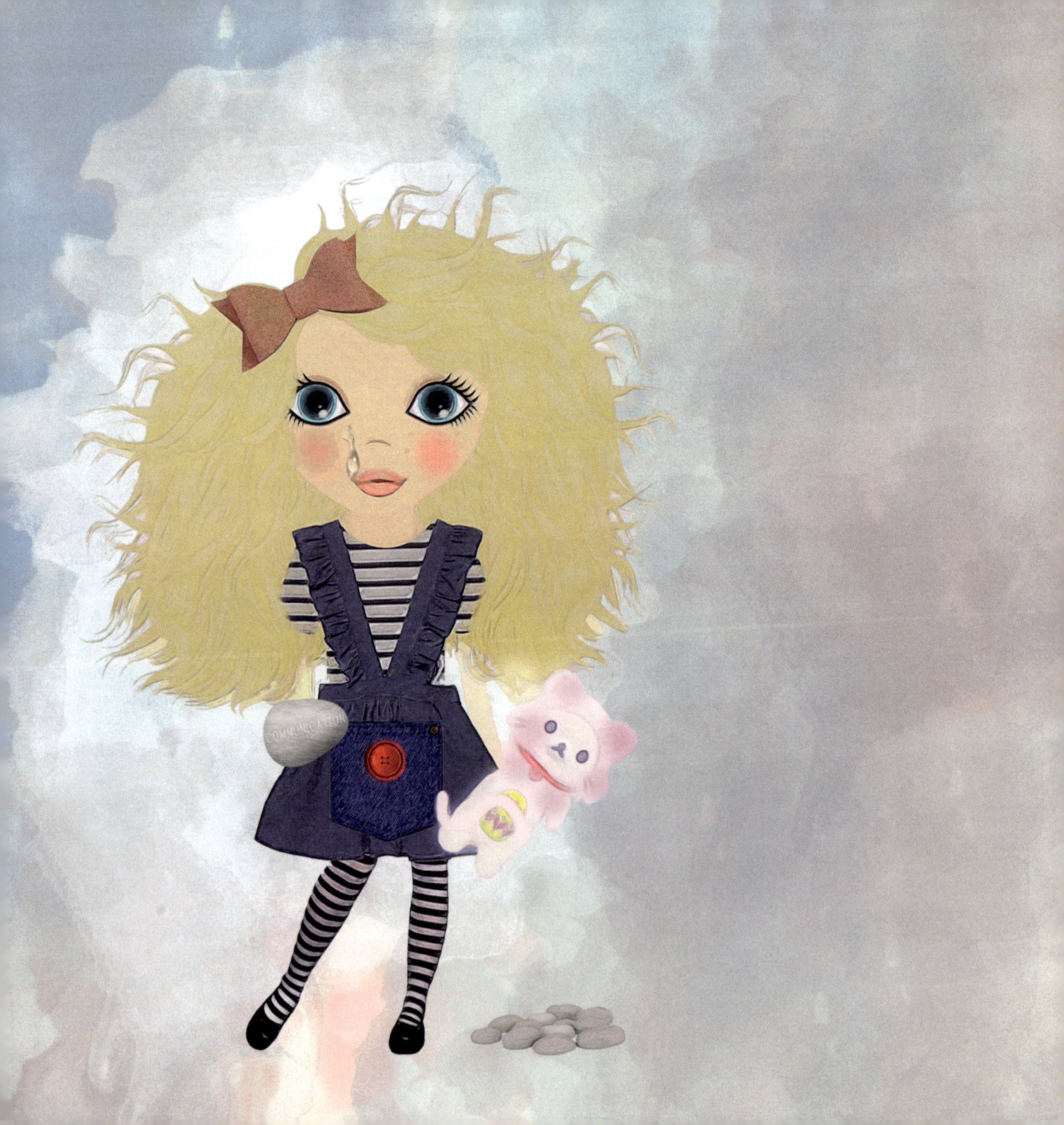
COMMUNICATION

BUT this made the other children think she was odd.

They didn't want to spend time with her.

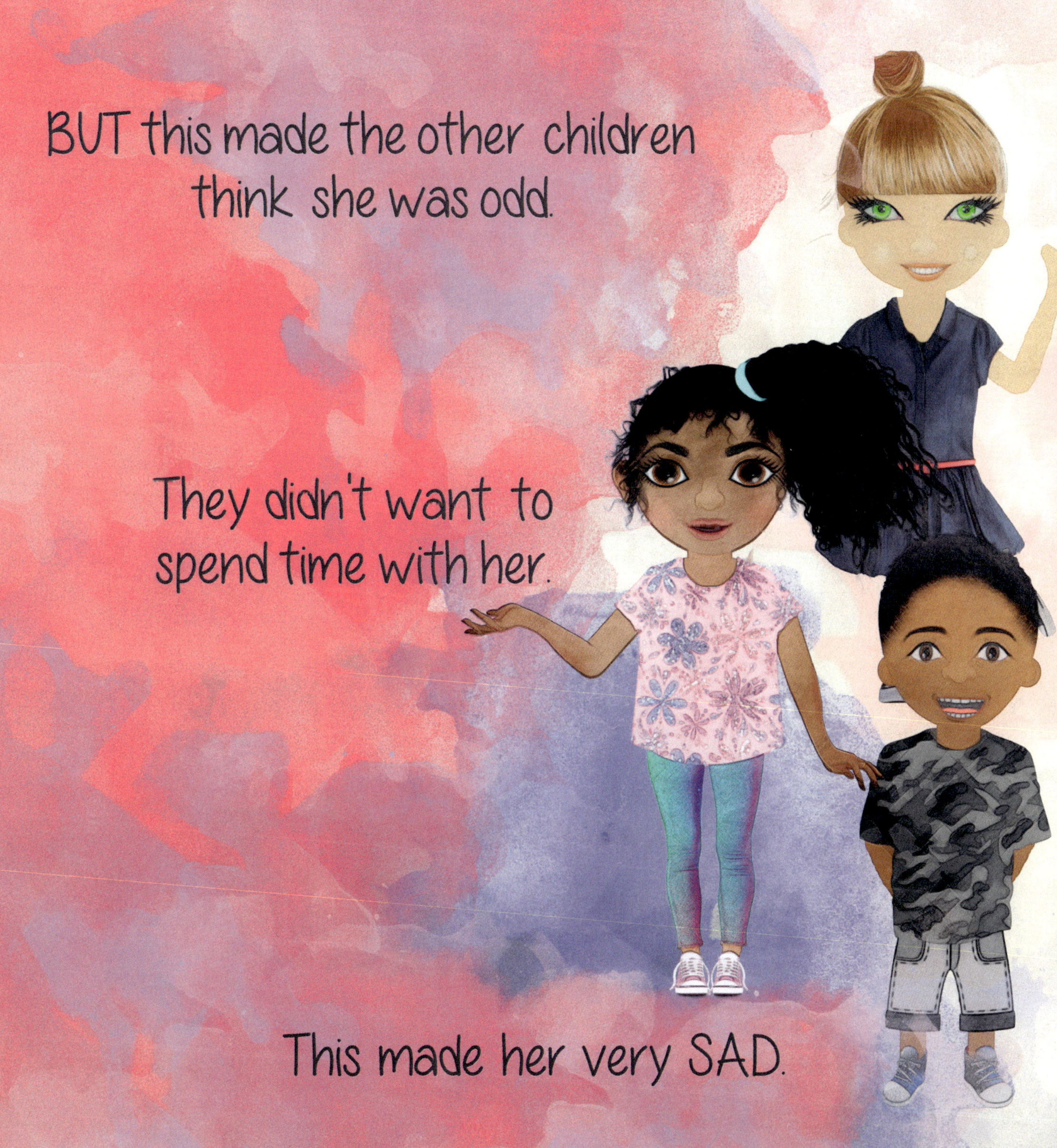

This made her very SAD.

She would love to have lots of friends to play with at school but her hidden secret made it difficult.

Her secret made her very honest. If she had a friend over and got tired, she would ask, "When are you going home?" which made her friend think she was rude.

If only the other children could learn her secret they would see what a loyal friend she could be.

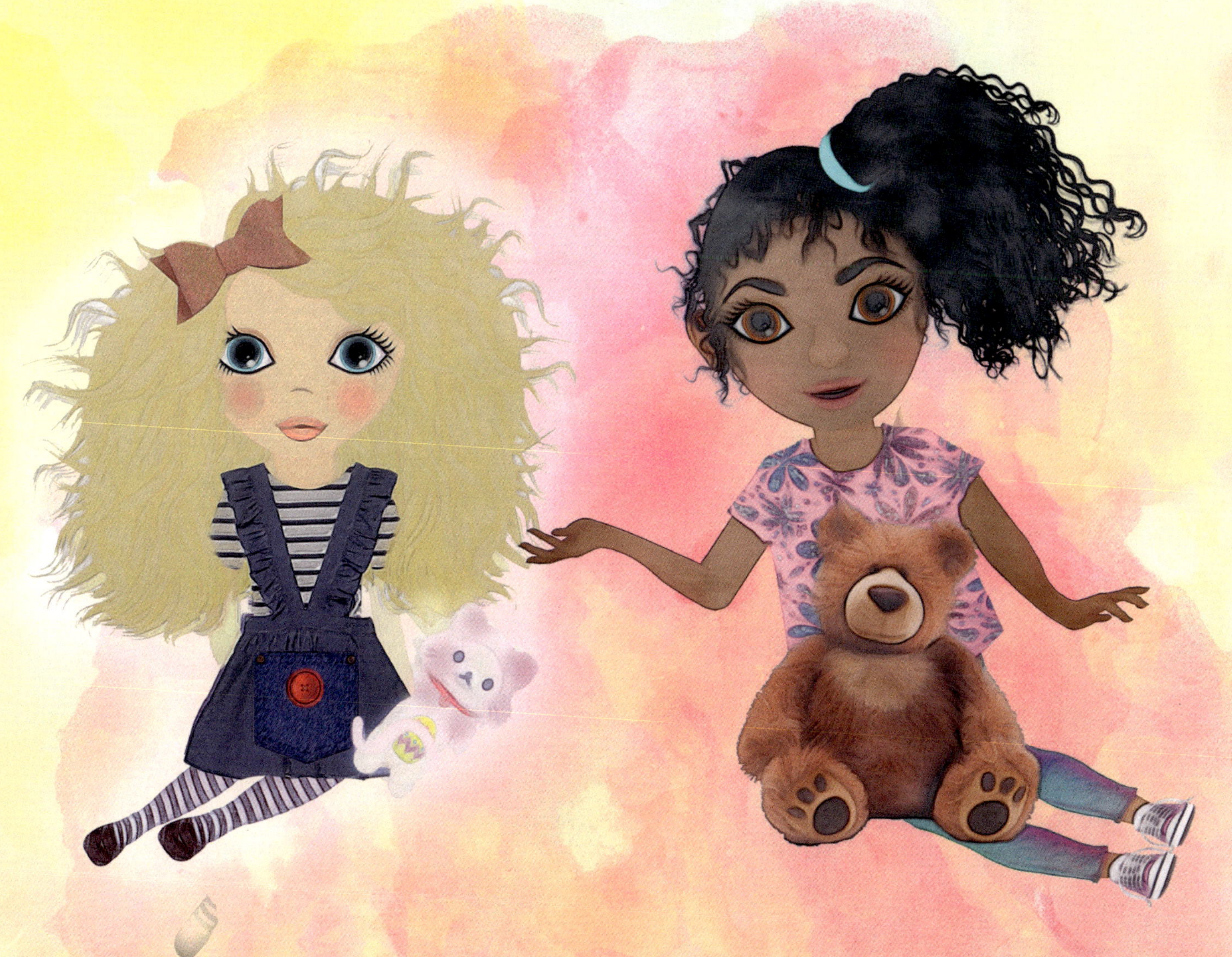

The little girl's teacher tried to nurture her secret, with lots of pictures of what was planned for the day and lots of praise, but, at times, he caused the little girl to become very anxious and stressed, unknowingly. The teacher would ask her questions and not give the little girl enough time to think.

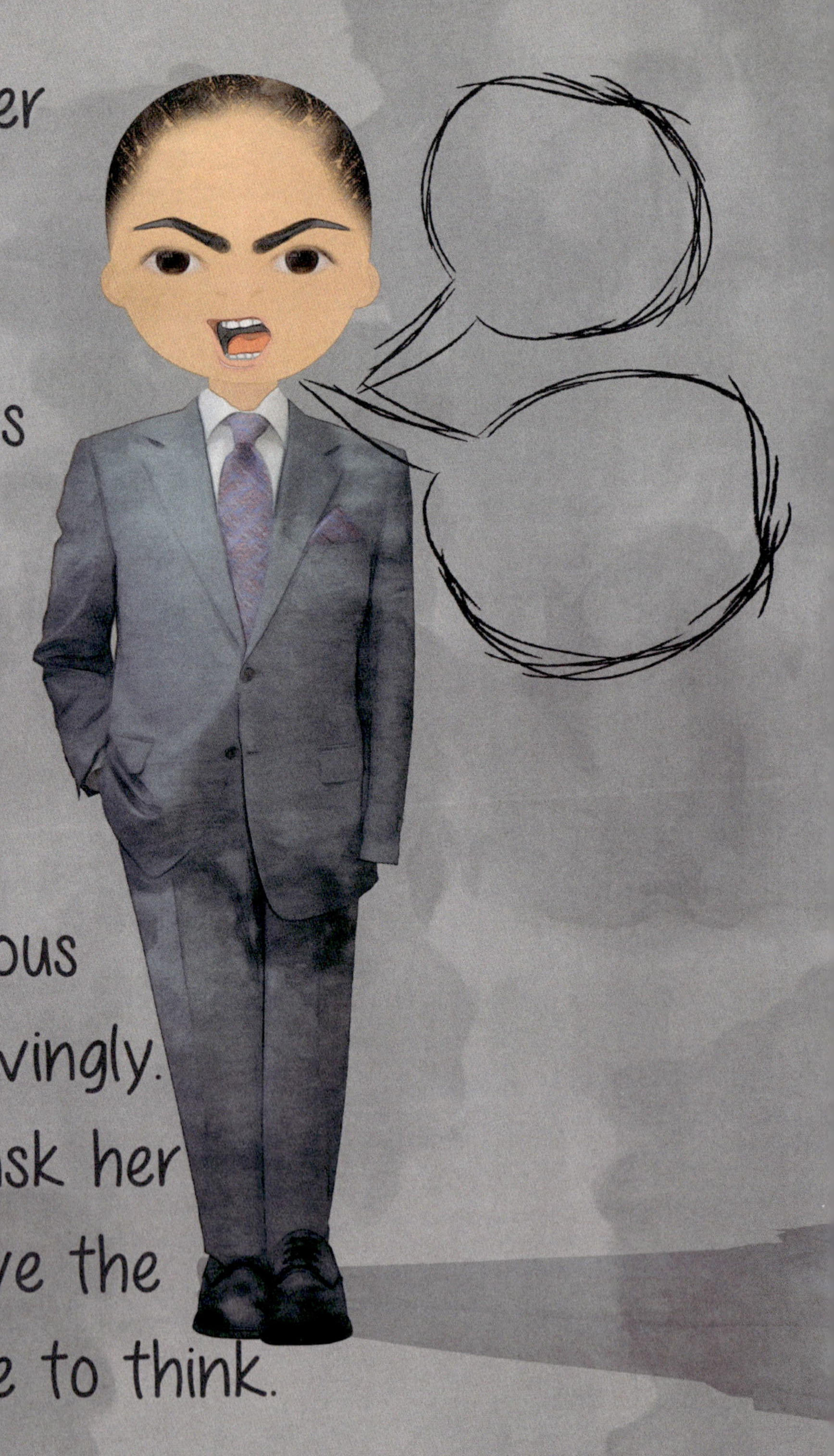

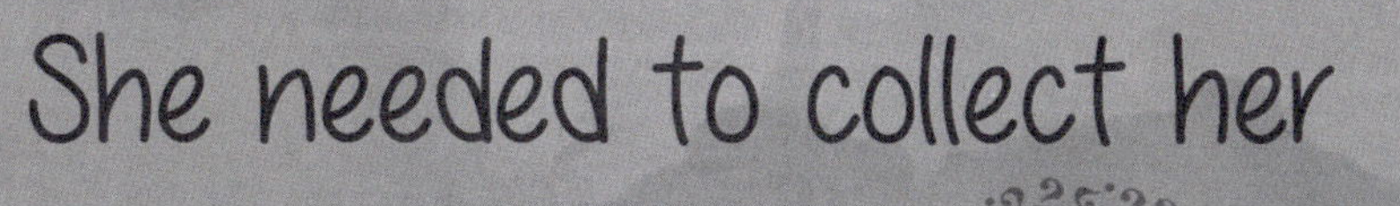

THOUGHTS

and reduce the anxiety that caused her to bite her nails until they BLED.

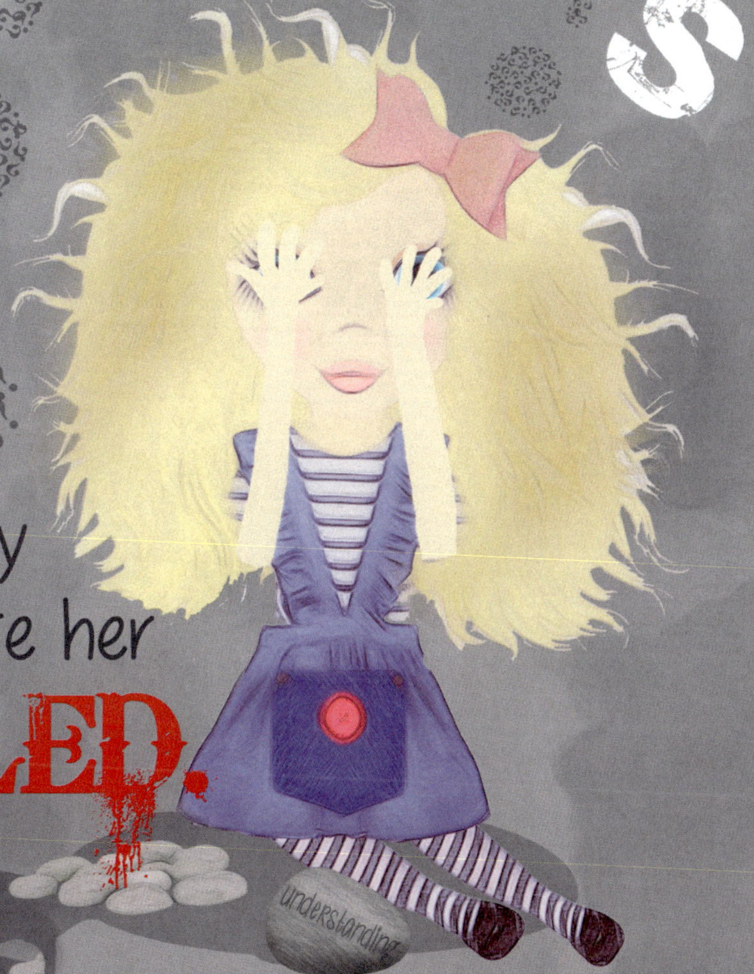

understanding

The little girl's secret also made her very literal. When the teacher said:

EVERYBODY SIT DOWN
NO ONE GET OUT OF THEIR SEATS OR MAKE A SOUND

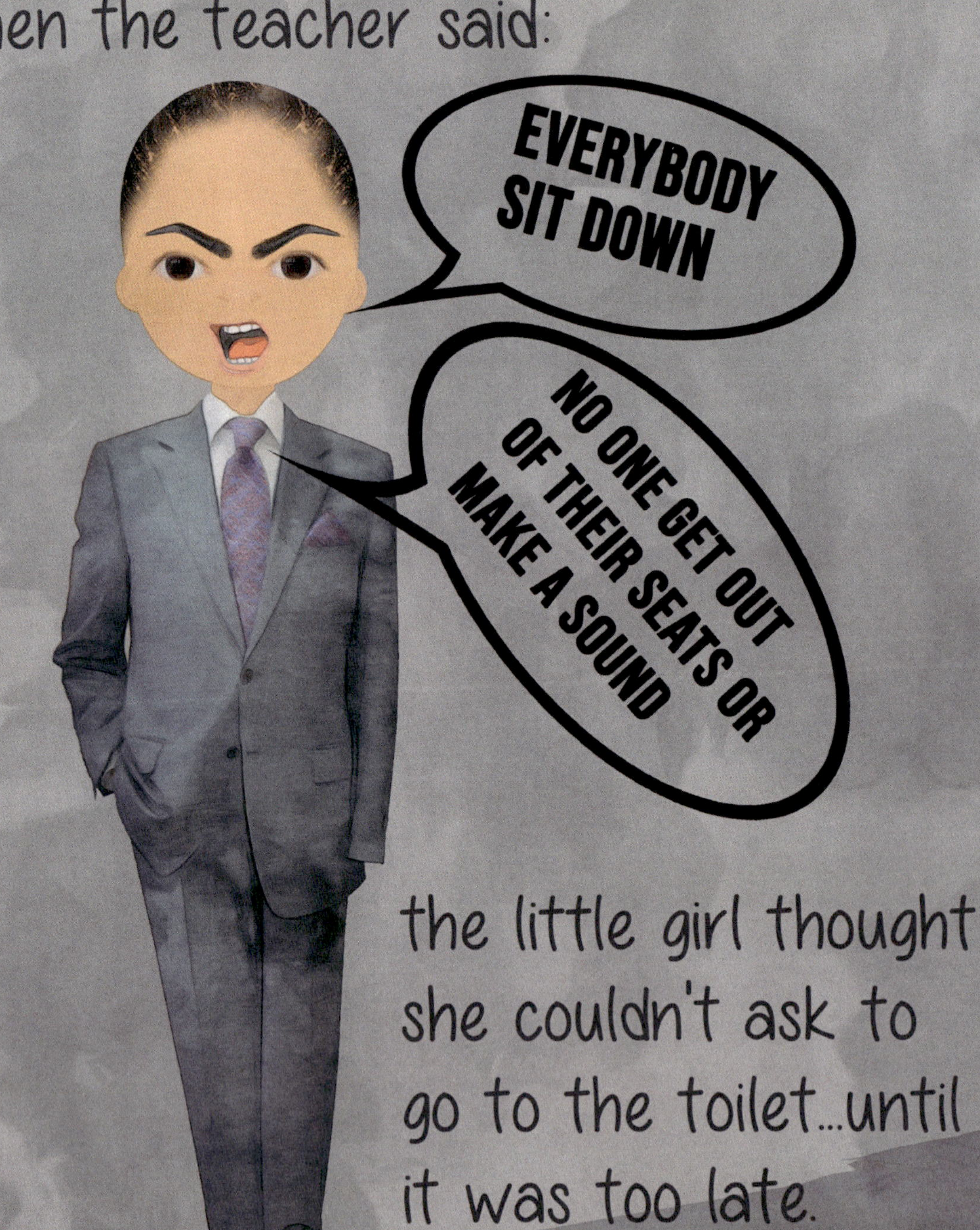

the little girl thought she couldn't ask to go to the toilet...until it was too late.

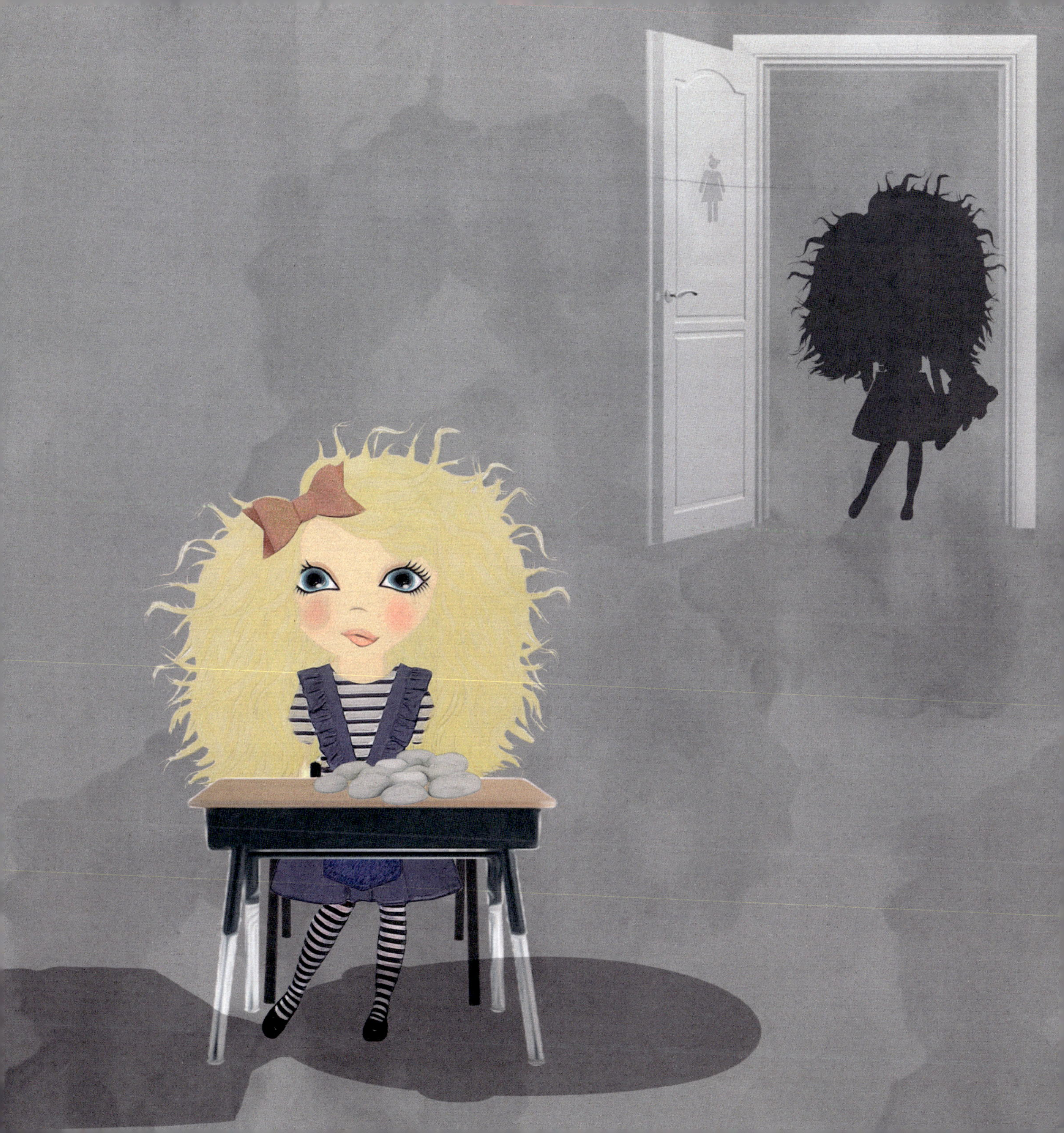

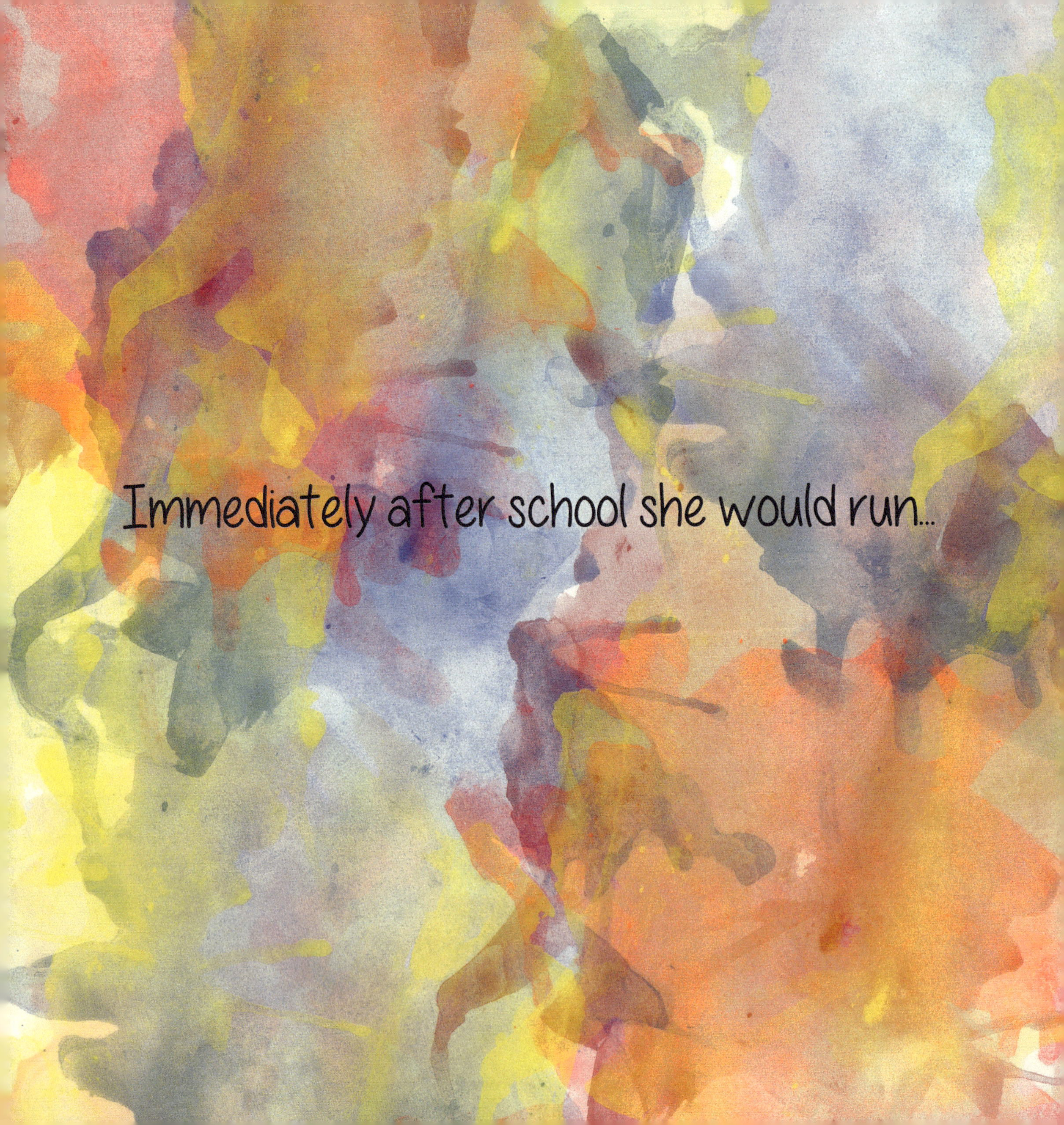

Immediately after school she would run...

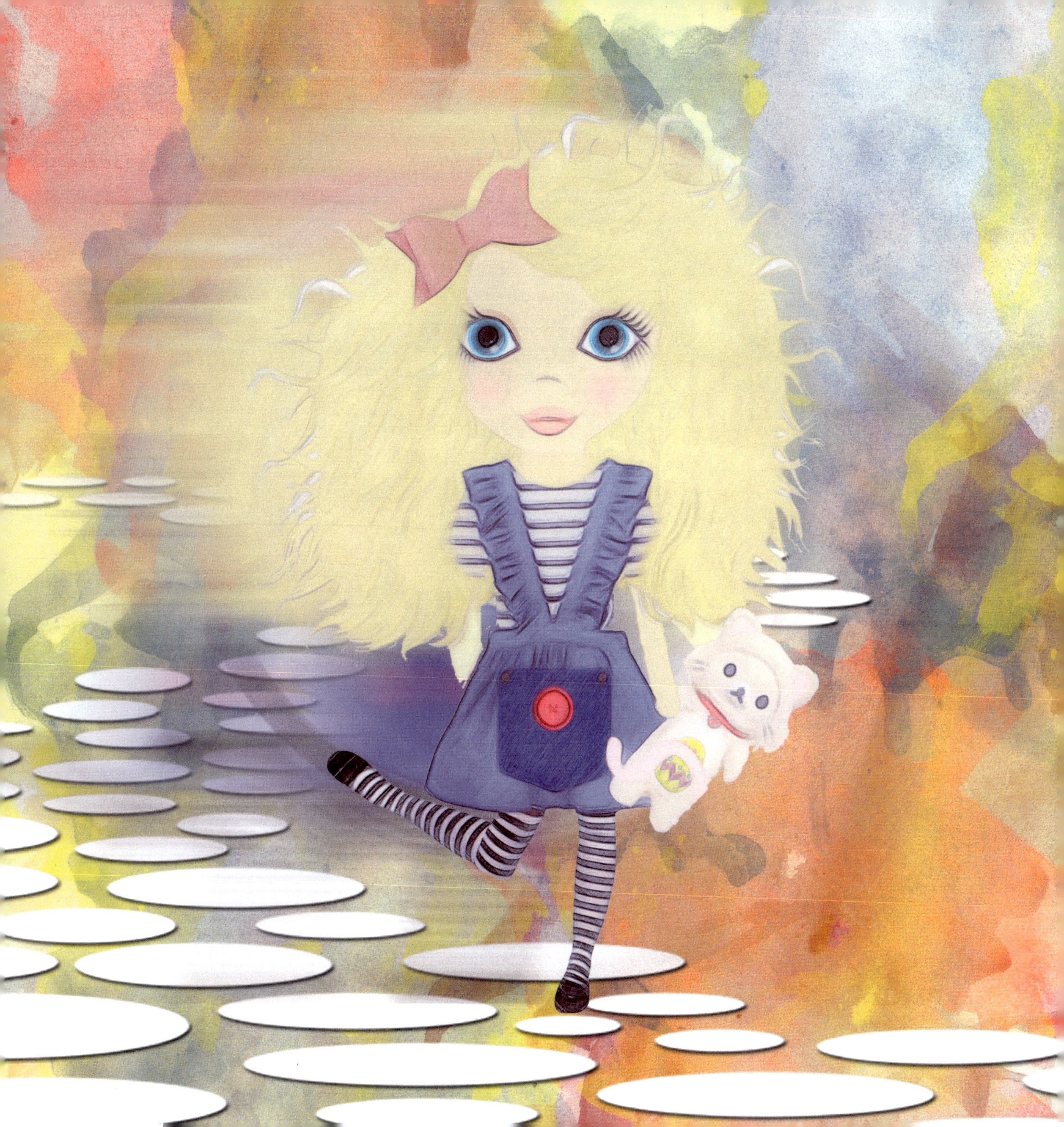

to give her mummy a hug, knowing
Mummy held the key to her happiness.

Mummy knew not to ask
about her day.

She just let her be herself again

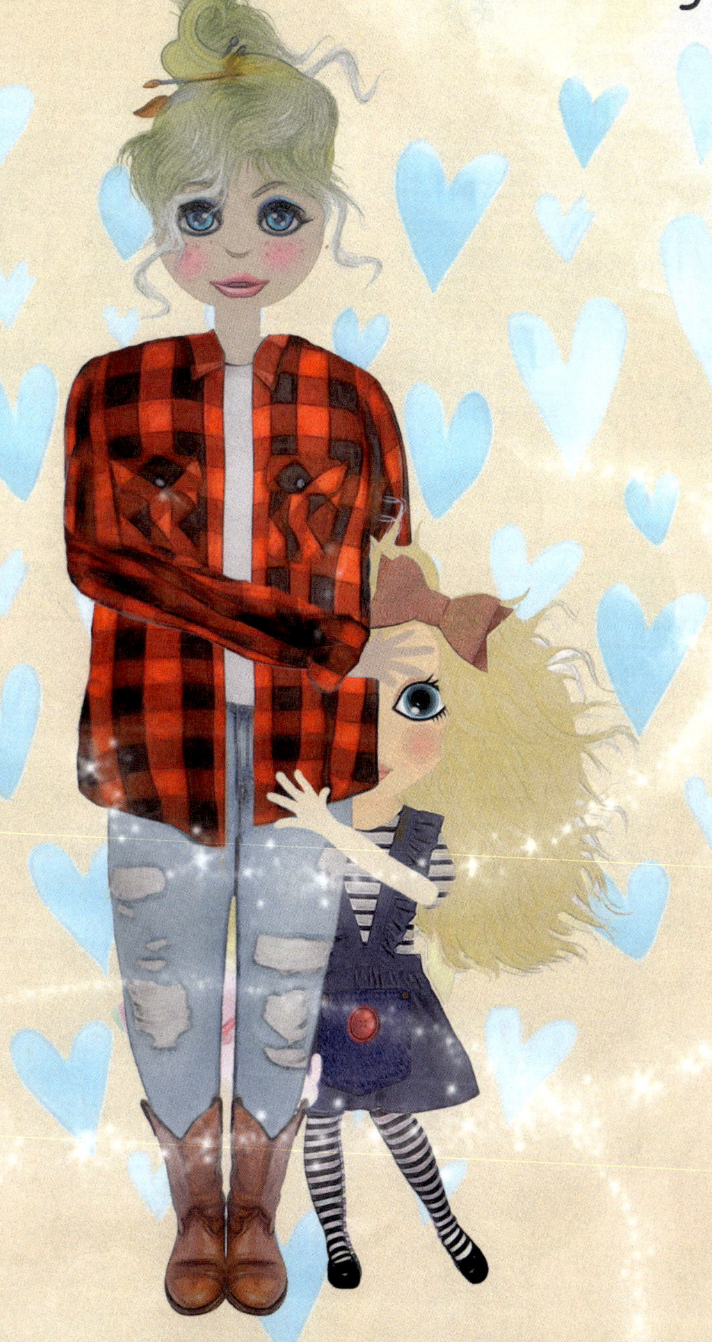

in her own safe surroundings.

When the little girl asked to suck her dummy in the car after school, Mummy gave it to her without judgement.

She knew it was the quickest way to settle the little girl's whirlpool of emotions.

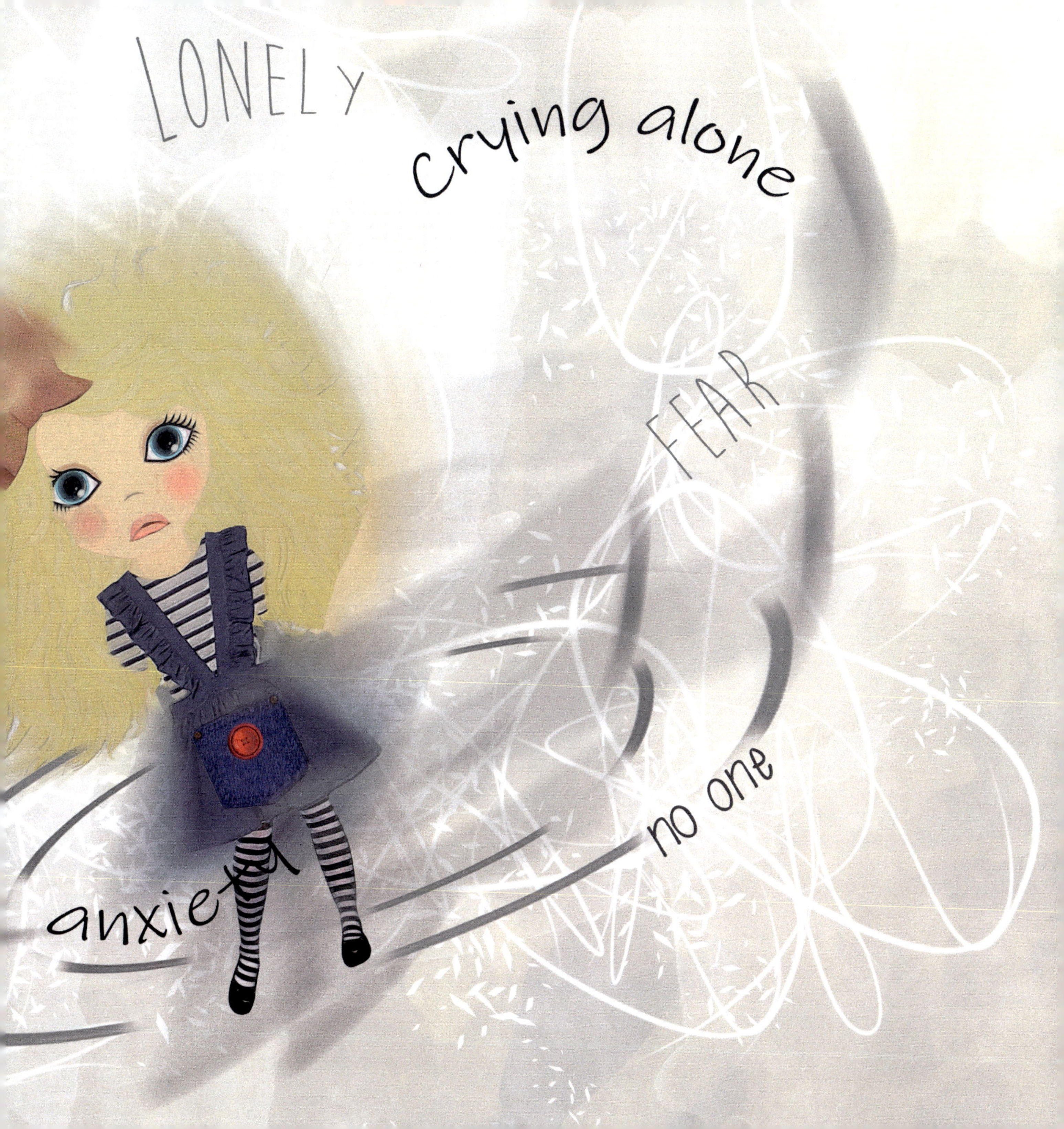

LONELY

crying alone

FEAR

no one

anxiety

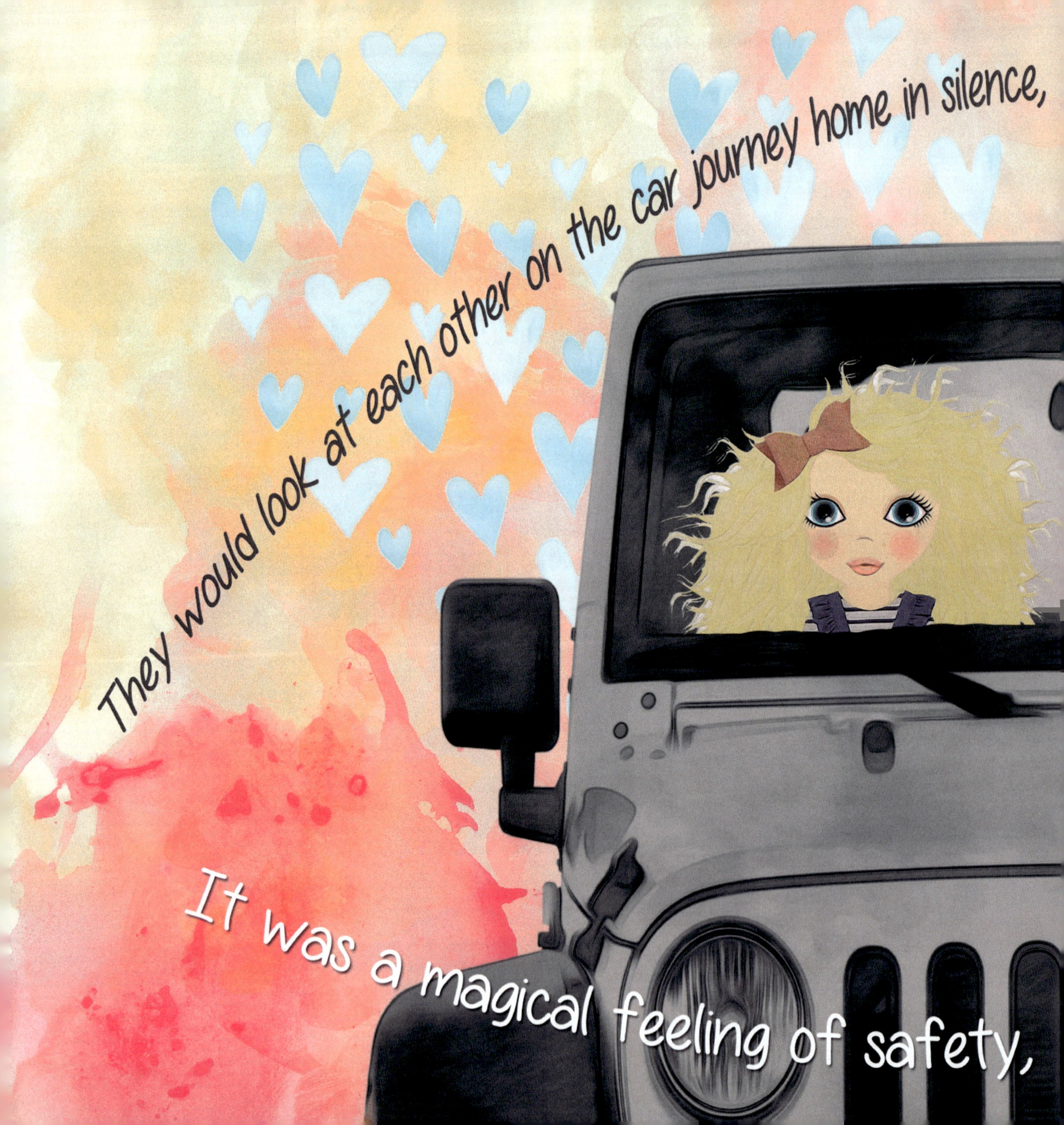

They would look at each other on the car journey home in silence,

It was a magical feeling of safety,

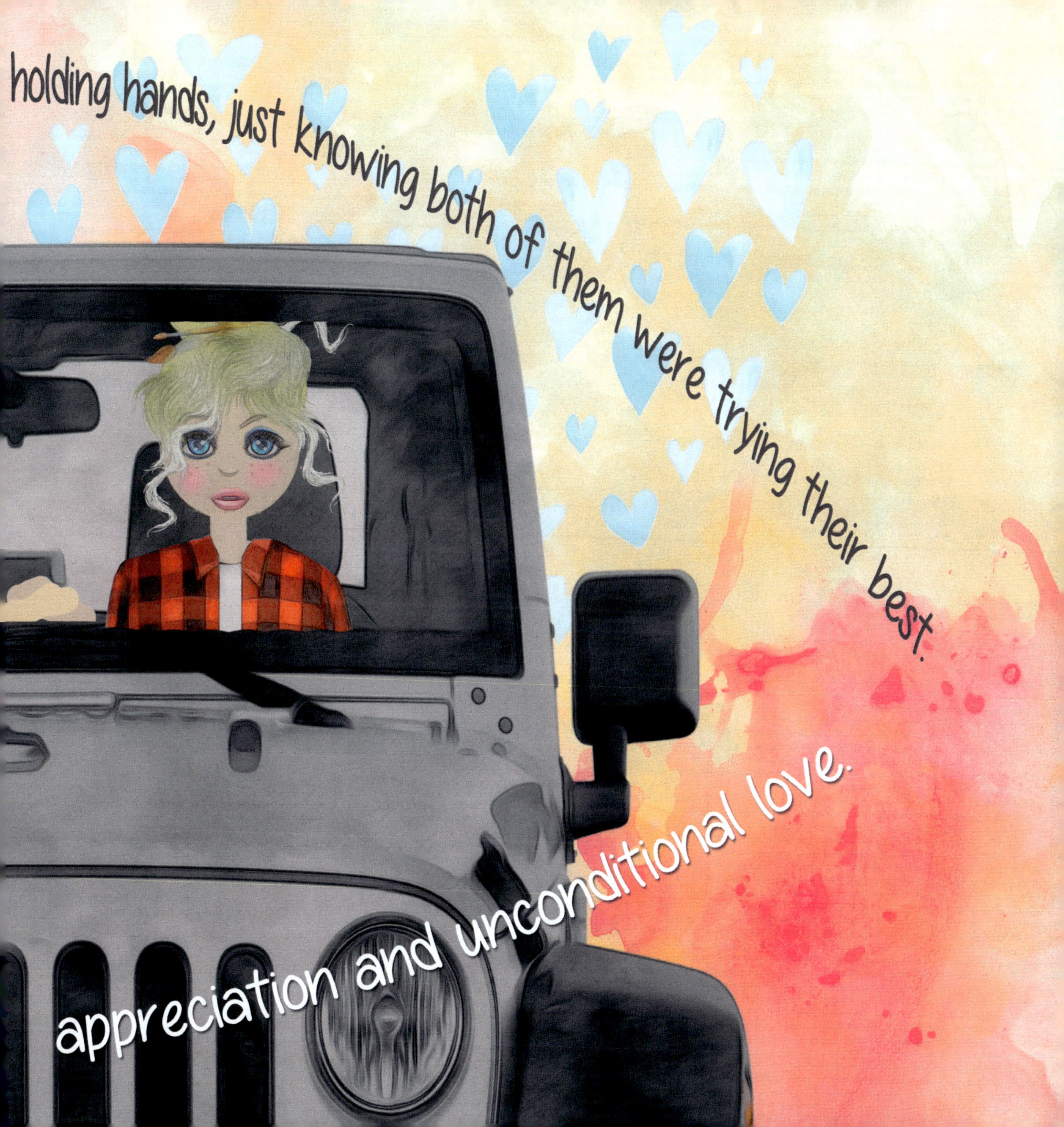

holding hands, just knowing both of them were trying their best.

appreciation and unconditional love.

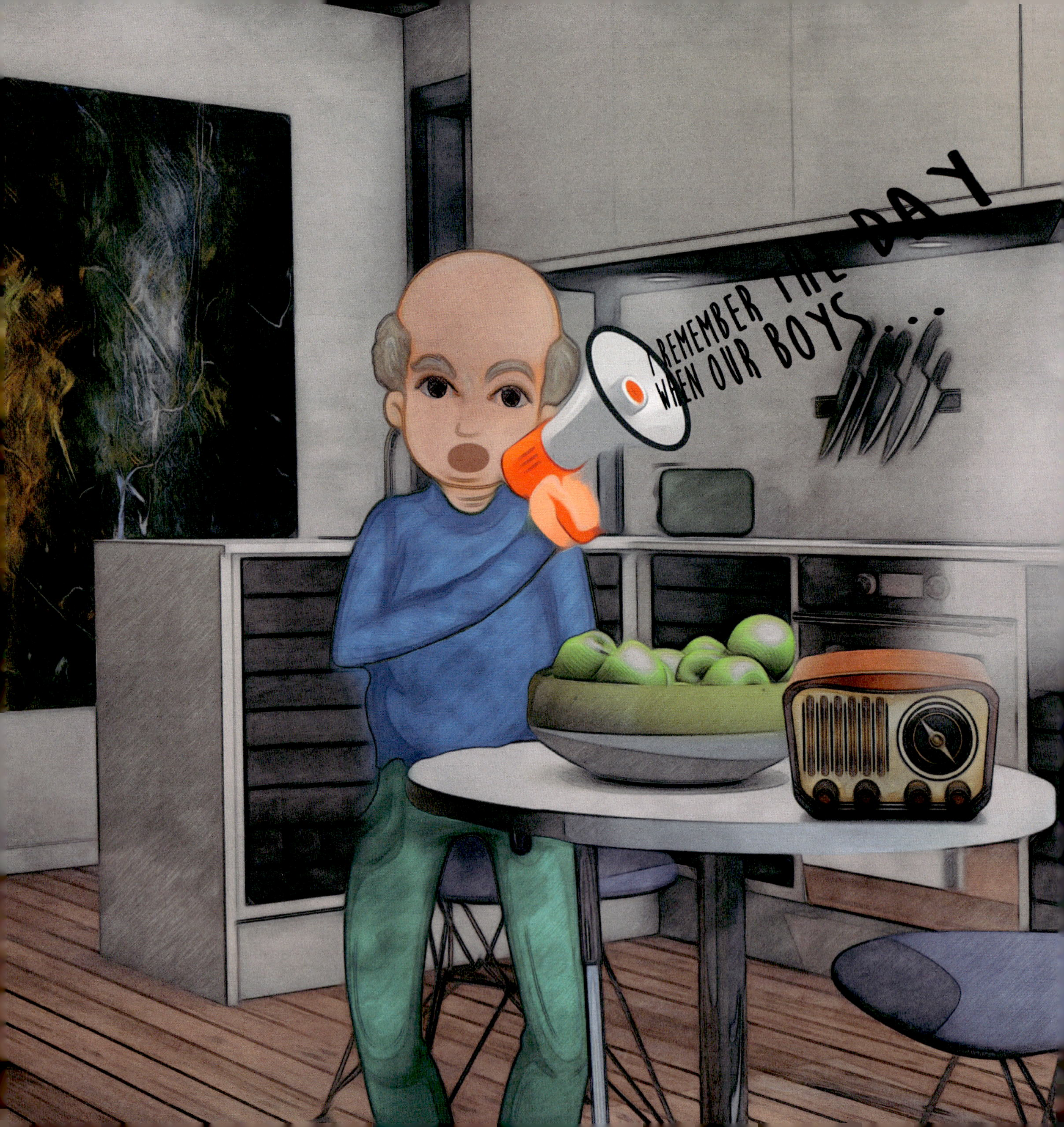
I REMEMBER THE DAY
WHEN OUR BOYS....

When she would visit her Grandma and Grandpa they would pretend they knew her secret... but they didn't.

Grandpa would talk REALLY LOUDLY and the little girl's secret told her to go into another room and shut the door or to cover her ears.

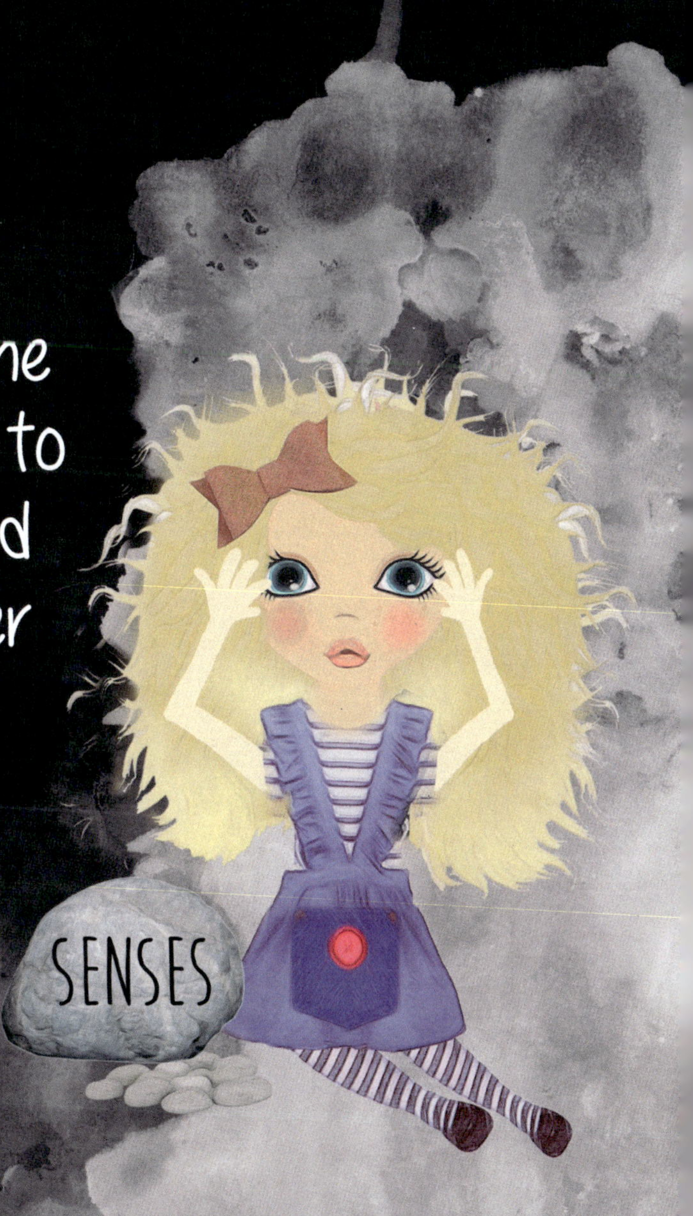

Grandma would make stew for dinner but the little girl's secret played tricks on her senses - it made the stew look like a bowl of

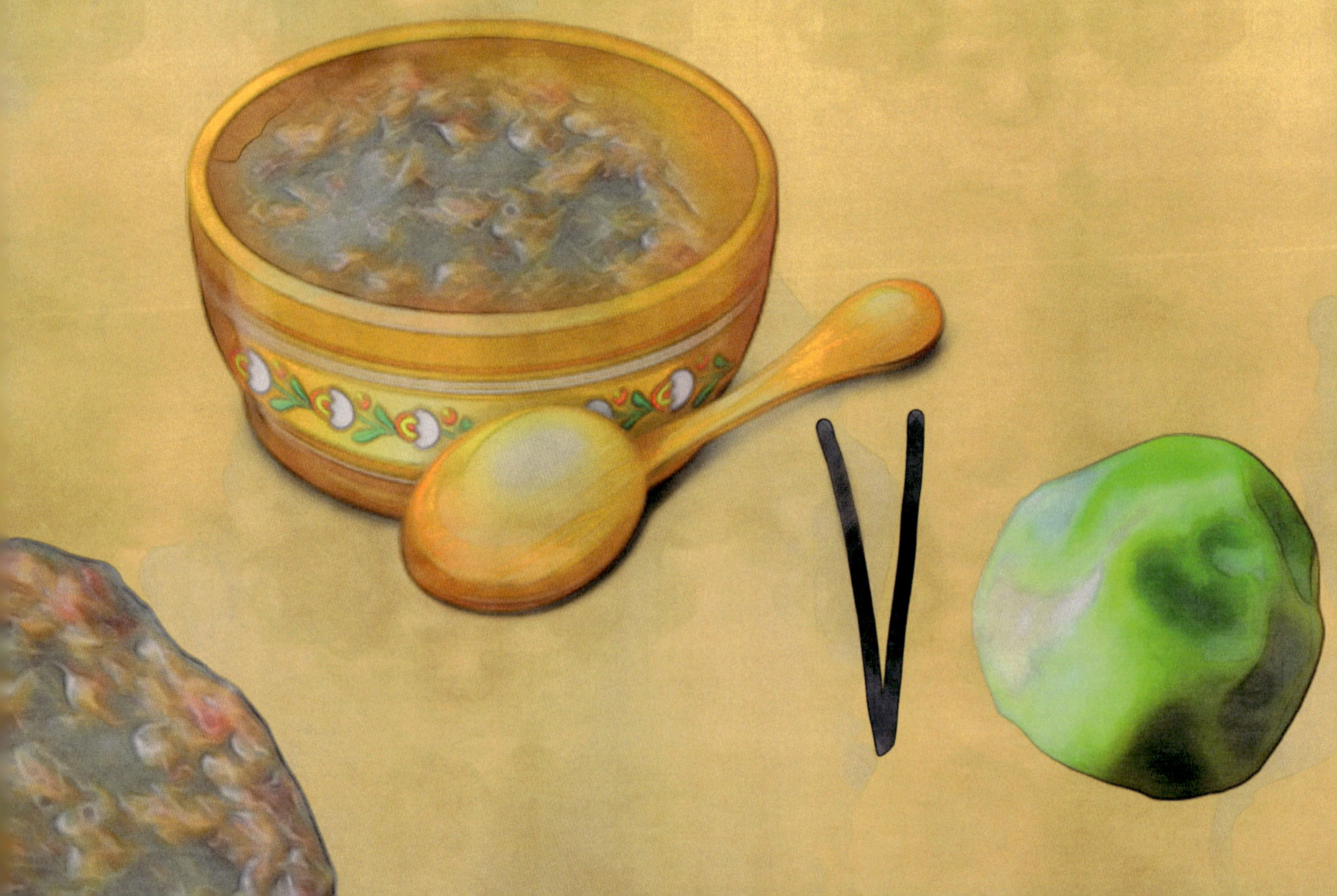

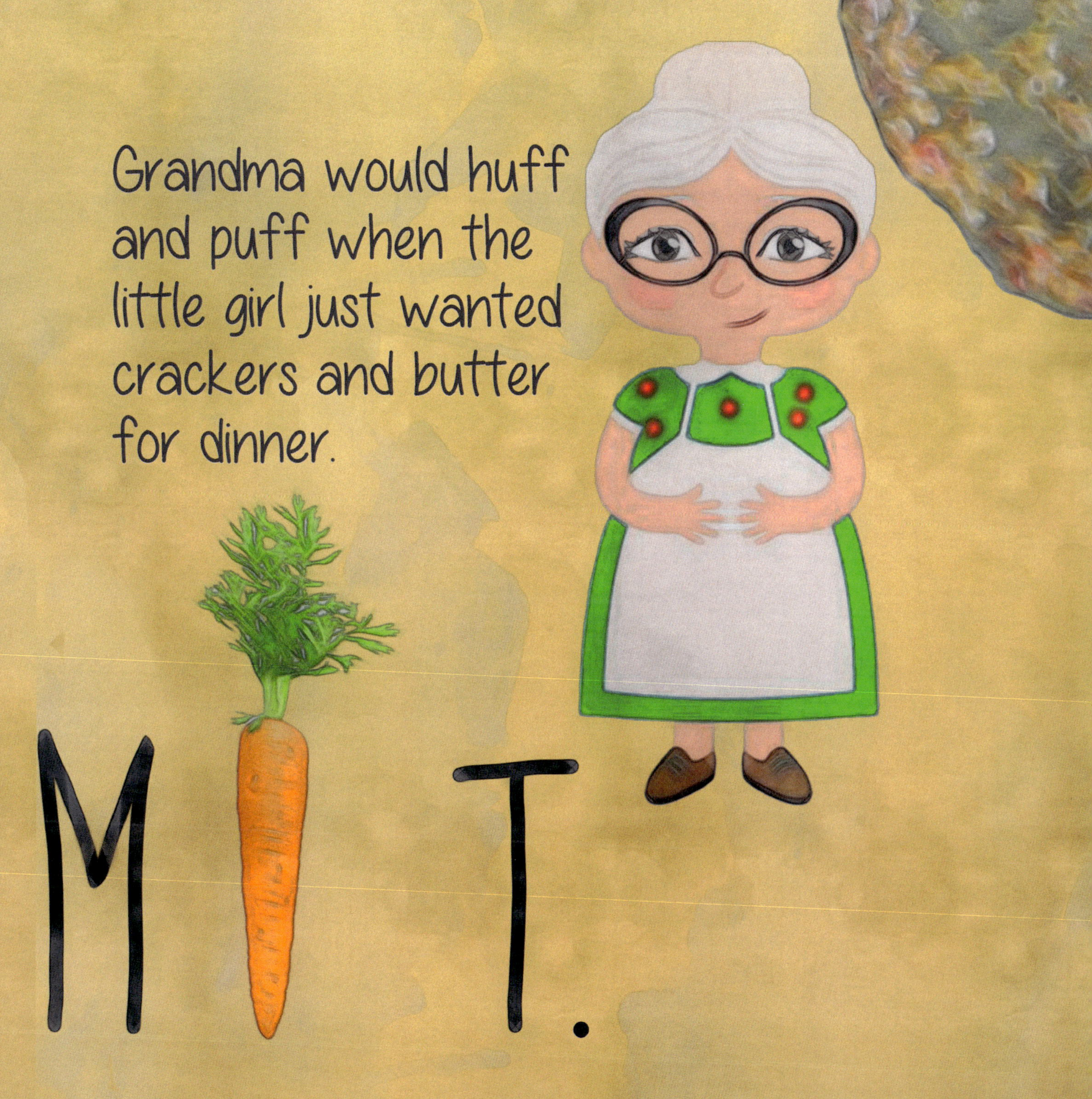
Grandma would huff
and puff when the
little girl just wanted
crackers and butter
for dinner.

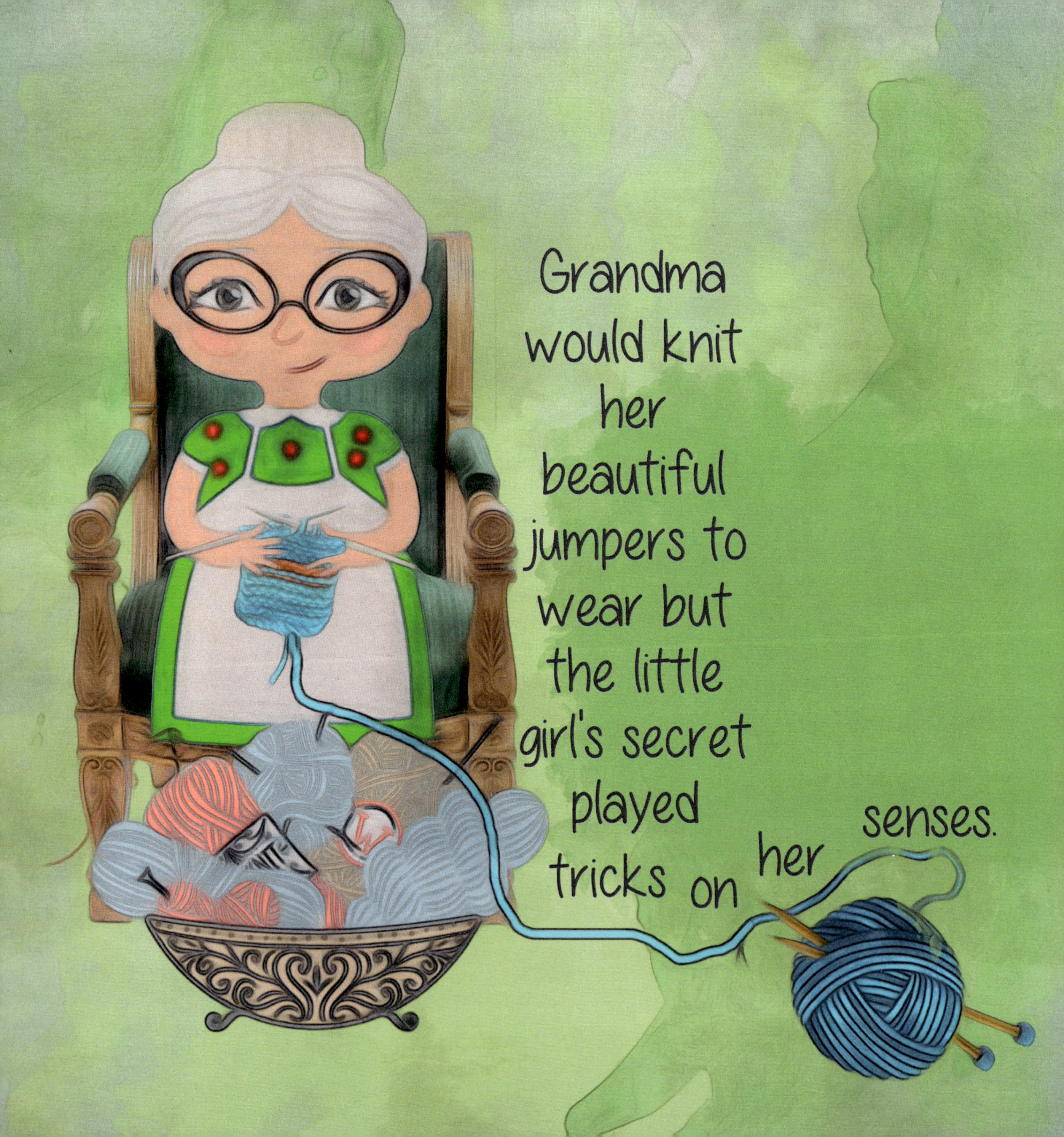
Grandma would knit her beautiful jumpers to wear but the little girl's secret played tricks on her senses.

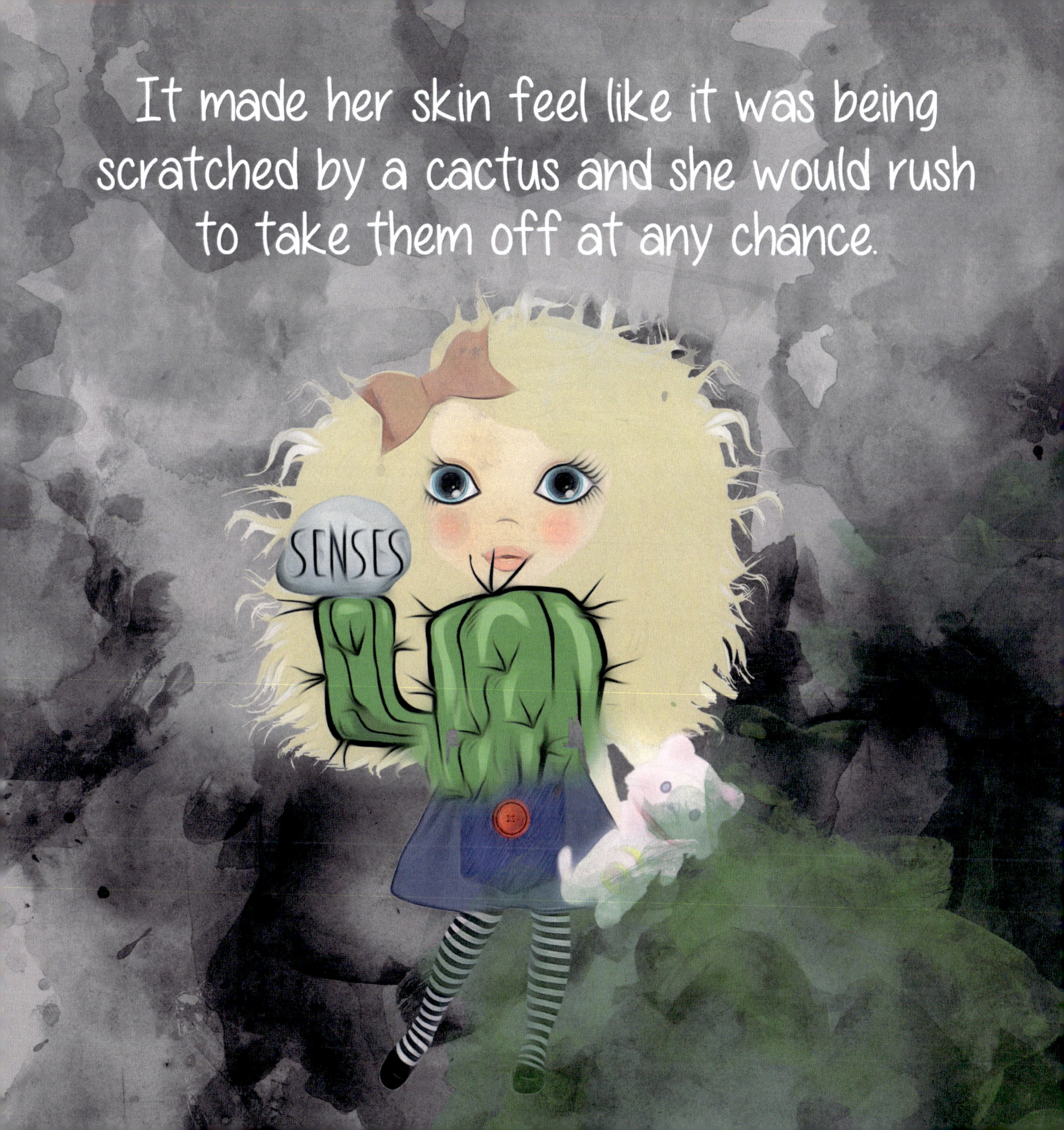
It made her skin feel like it was being scratched by a cactus and she would rush to take them off at any chance.

Grandma loved to brush the little girl's hair and couldn't understand why the little girl would cry so much.

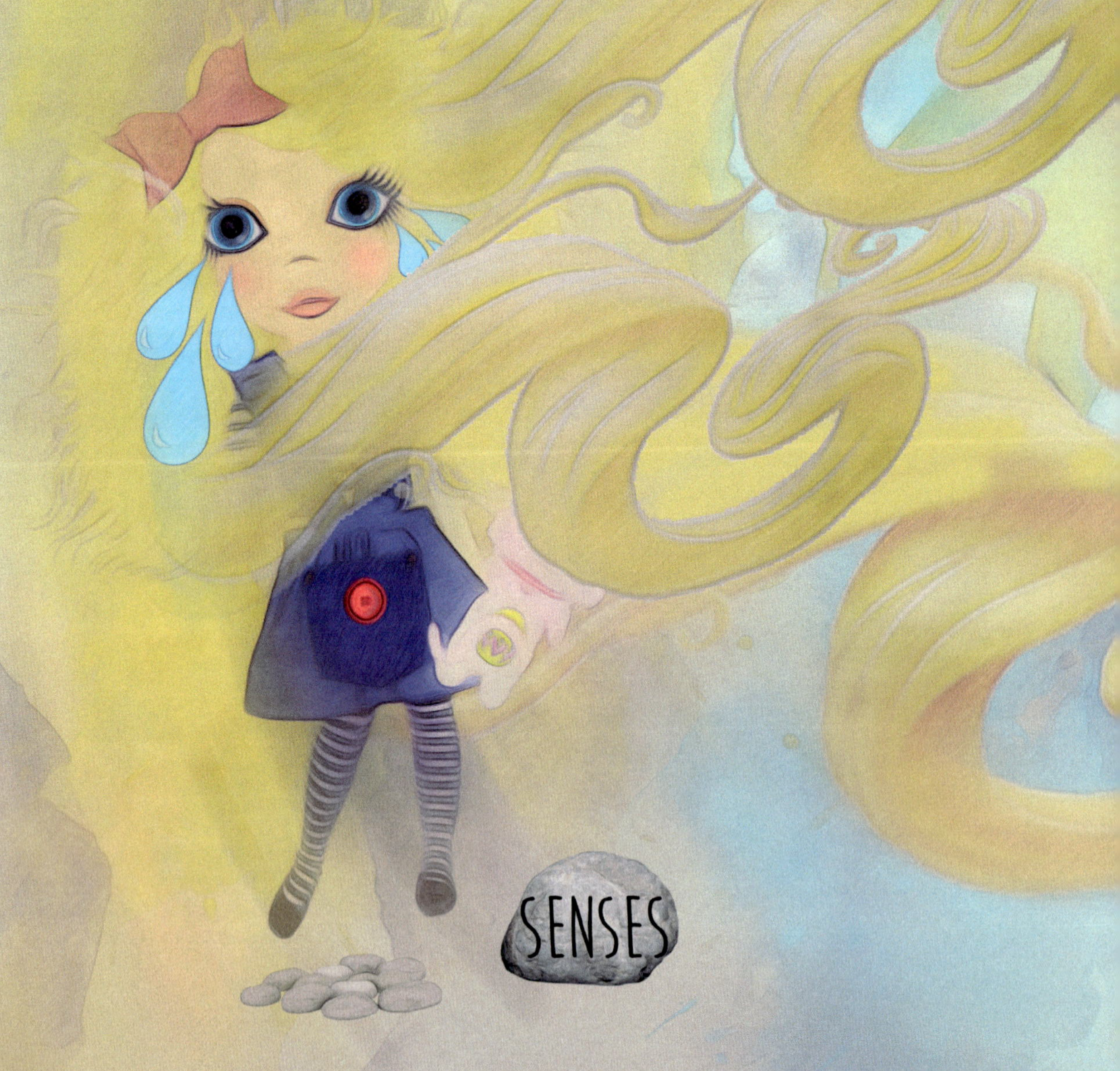

It was the little girl's secret again, making her feel like she was getting swung around by her hair.

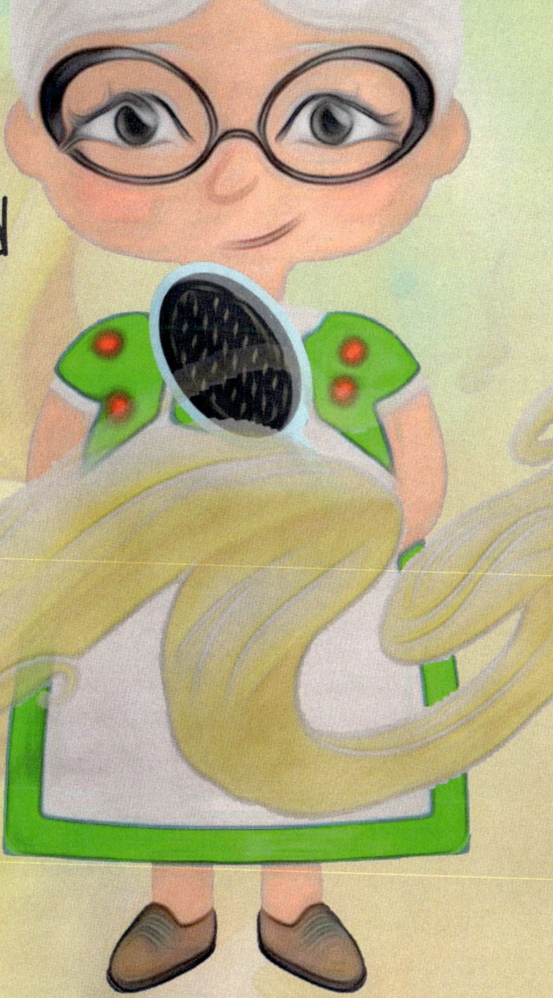

The little girl would talk about the same set of toys endlessly until Grandma would take her to the toy shop to pick something new.

But, to the little girl, it seemed every toy had a fault or wasn't the exact brand she collected.

When Grandma suggested buying a replacement for her favourite pussycat, who was worn and tattered, only the original would do.

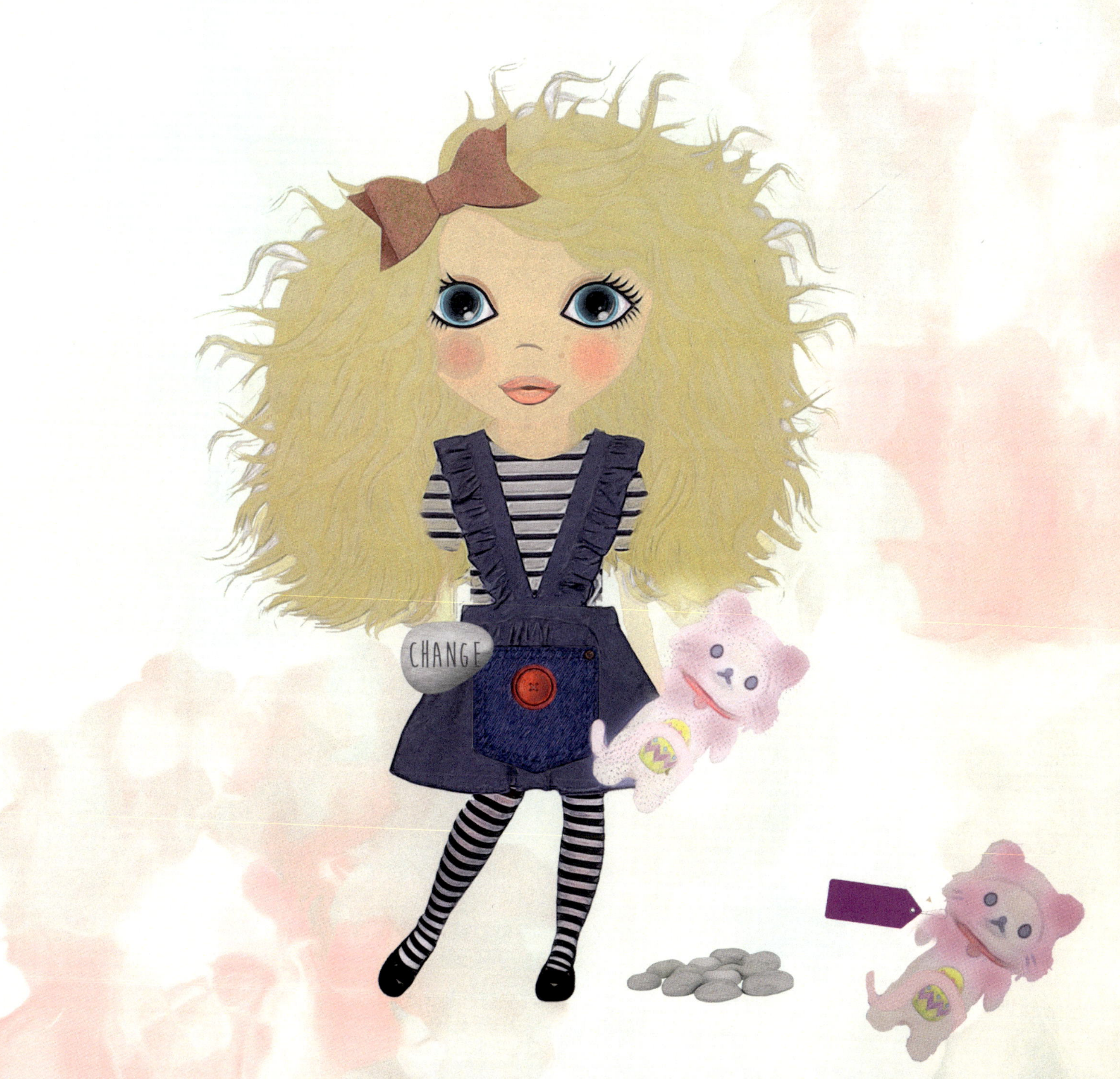
CHANGE

Grandpa and Grandma didn't fully understand the little girl's secret, but it made them even better Grandparents without them realising. The unusual things the little girl did made them laugh and they loved her even more for showing them a new view of the world.

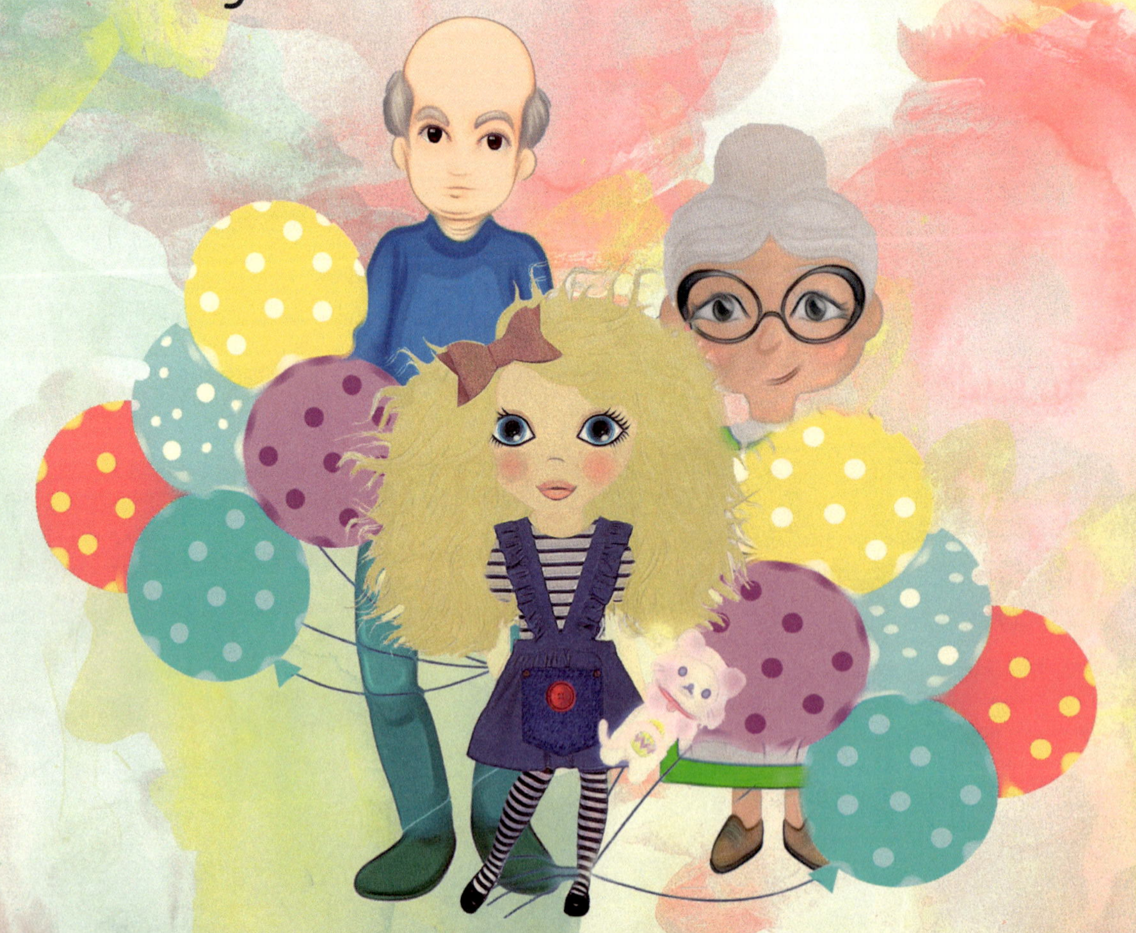

As the little girl got older she realised she had gathered a pocket bursting with pebbles that her secret had given her.

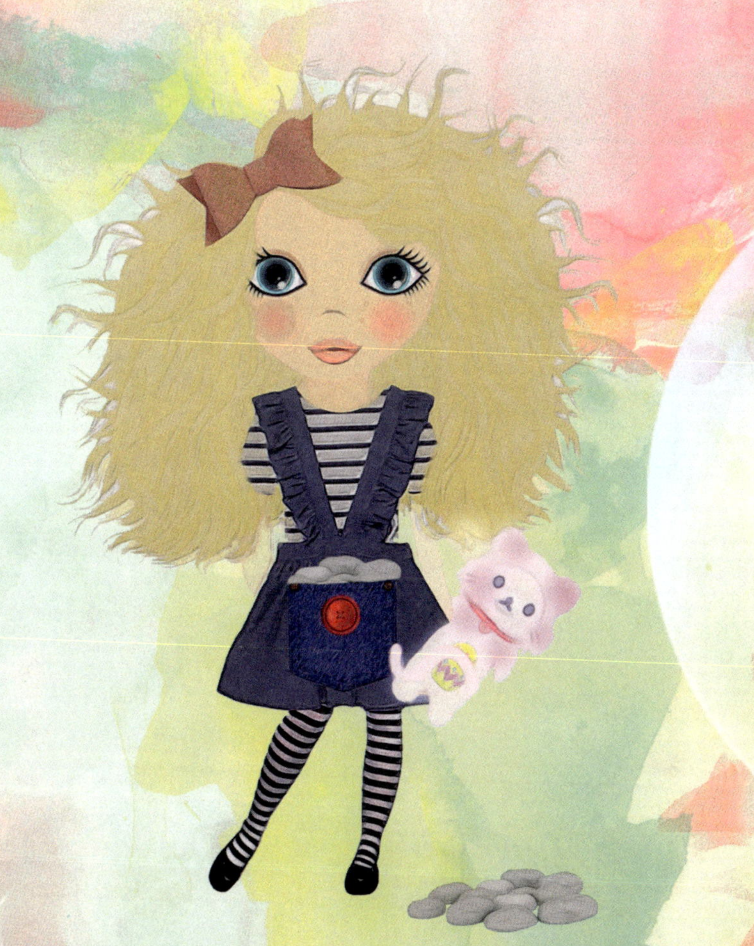

Each pebble told her something different, but she had no idea what they were for or why she even had them.

One day, the little girl and her mummy were doing her favourite thing - lining up her toys - but the little girl was struggling to carry her toys with the weight of her pocket of pebbles. It was even heavier now, bulging and overflowing, causing her great discomfort.

"What's wrong?"

Mummy asked, concerned.

Suddenly, the little girl flopped down onto the floor and the pebbles

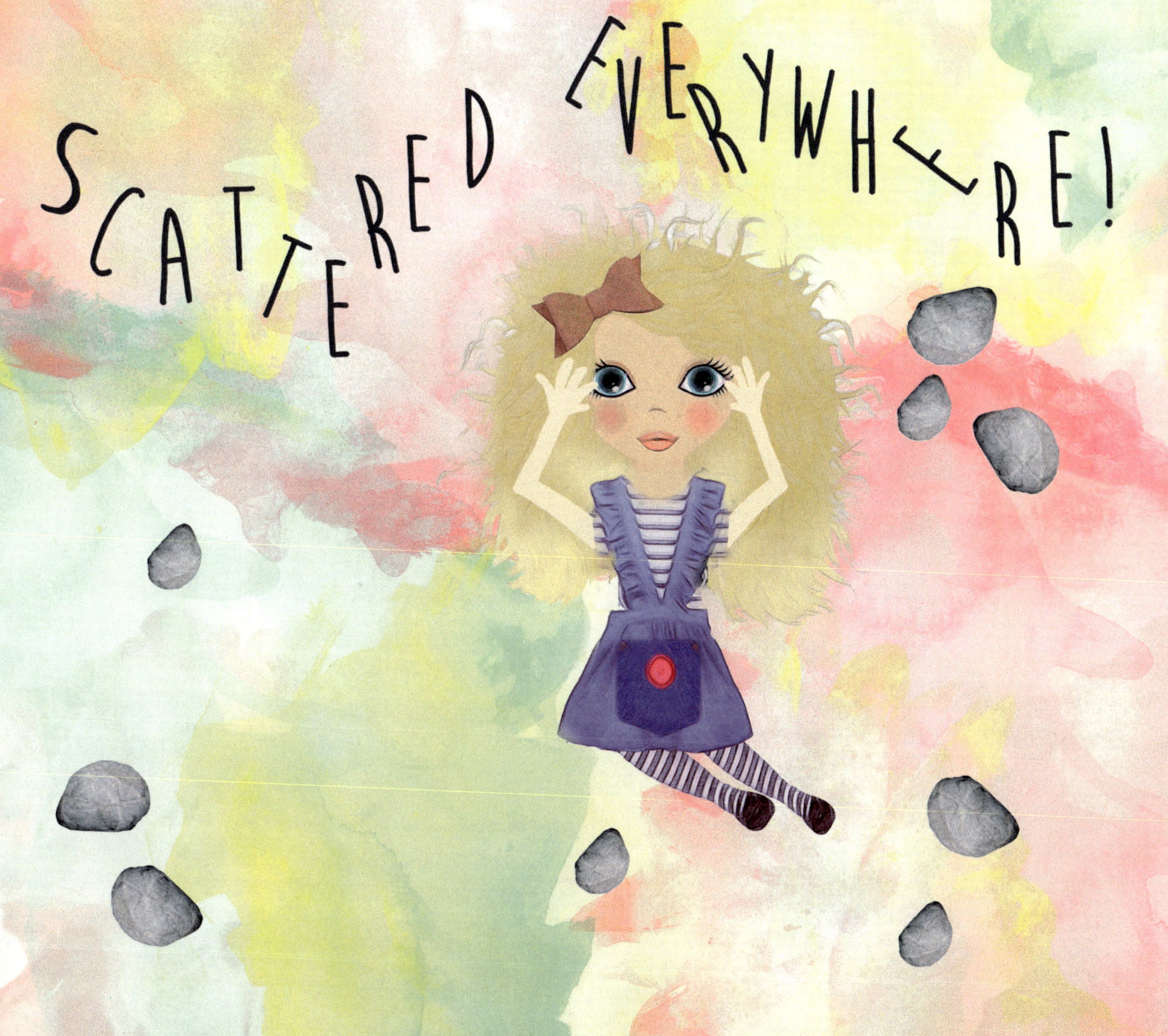

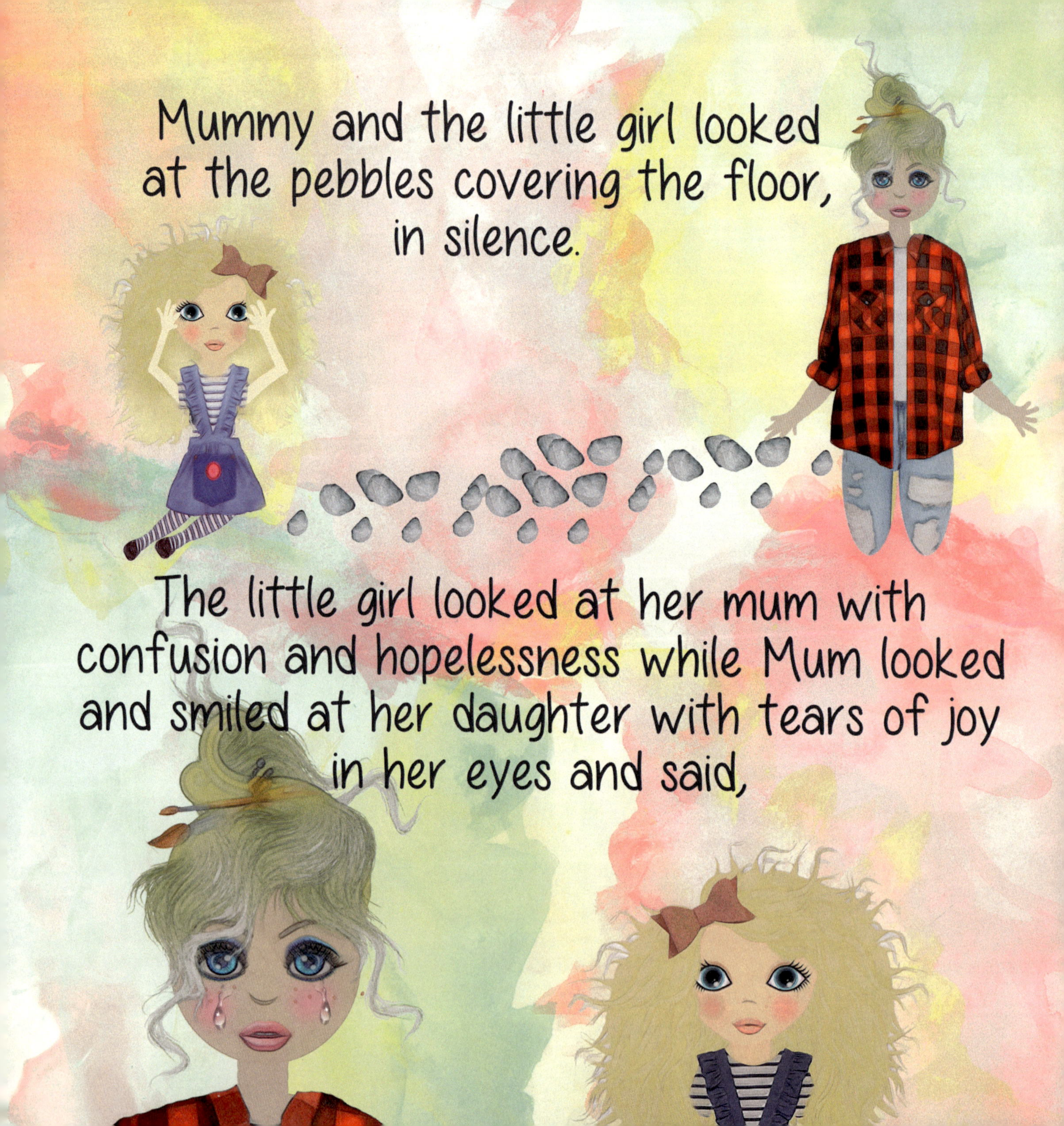

Mummy and the little girl looked at the pebbles covering the floor, in silence.

The little girl looked at her mum with confusion and hopelessness while Mum looked and smiled at her daughter with tears of joy in her eyes and said,

"Sweetheart, you have found all the clues you need for me to tell you your special secret. You are old enough now for me to share with you everything that makes me love you even more than I thought would ever be possible."

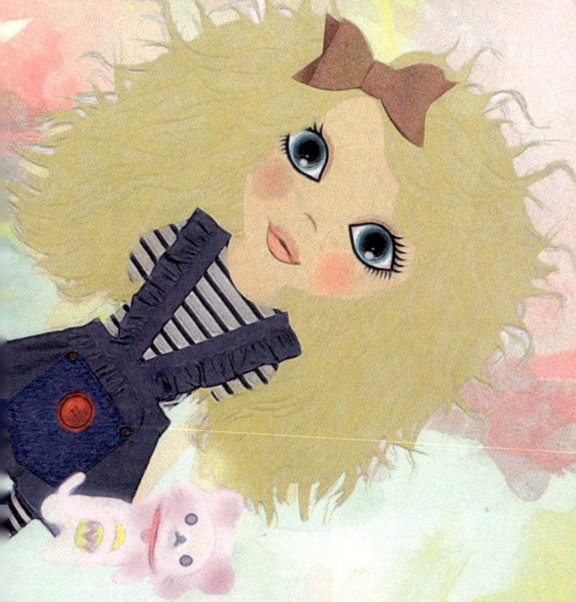

The confusion on the little girl's face remained,

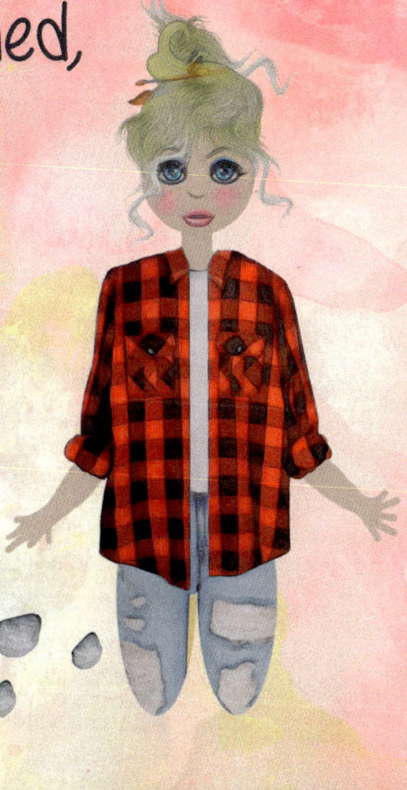

while Mum started to rearrange the pebbles on the floor.

They spelt...

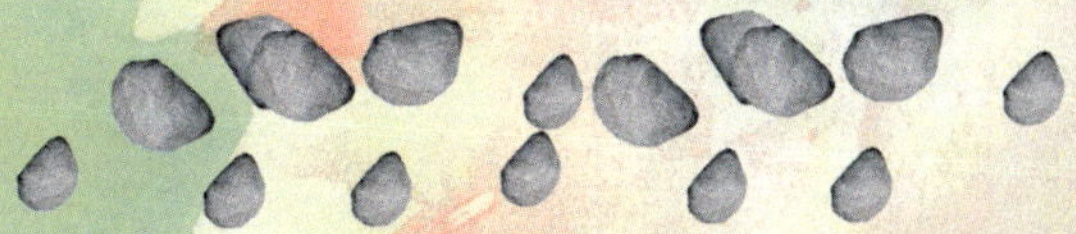

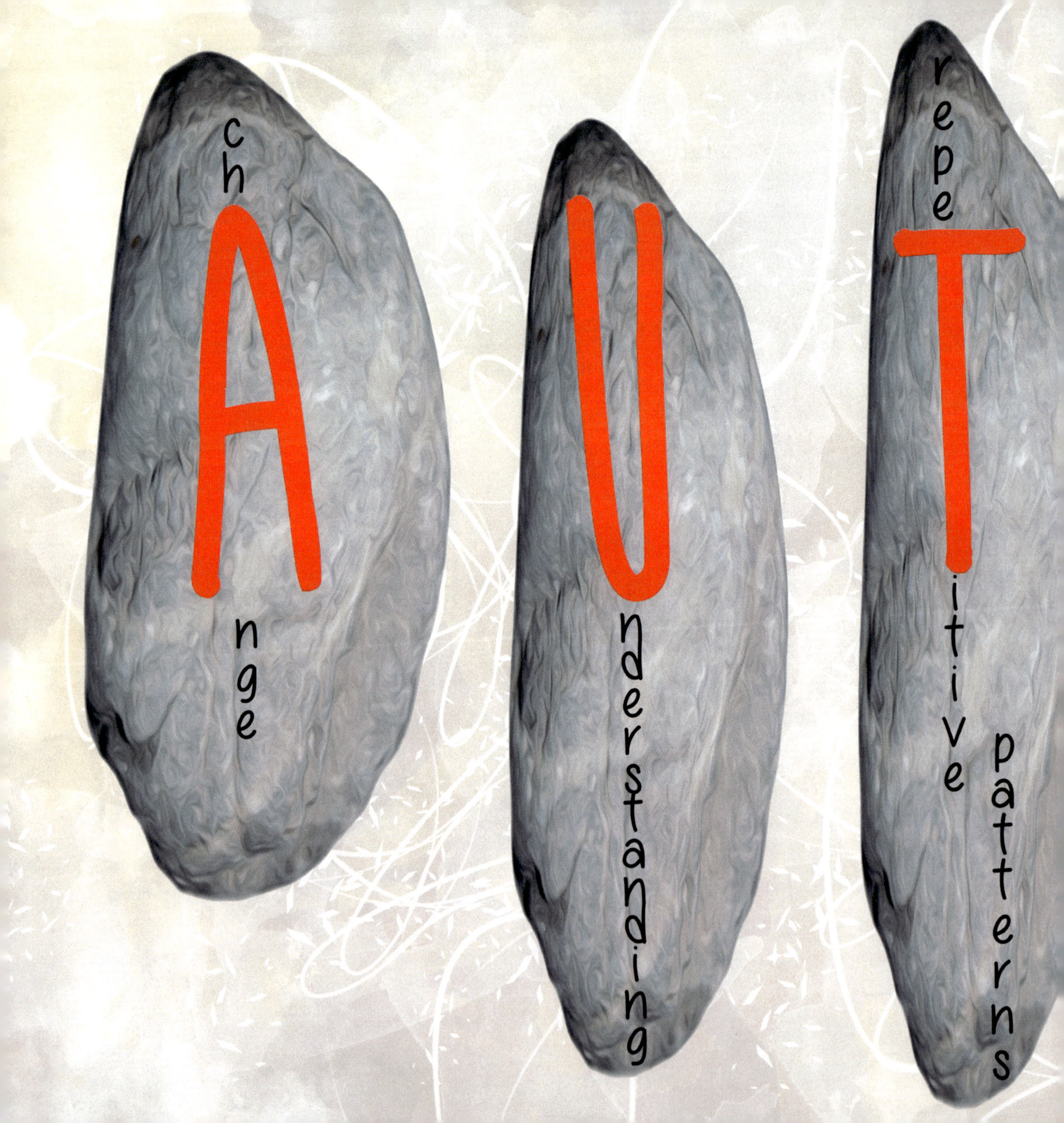

chAnge
Understanding
repeTitive
patterns

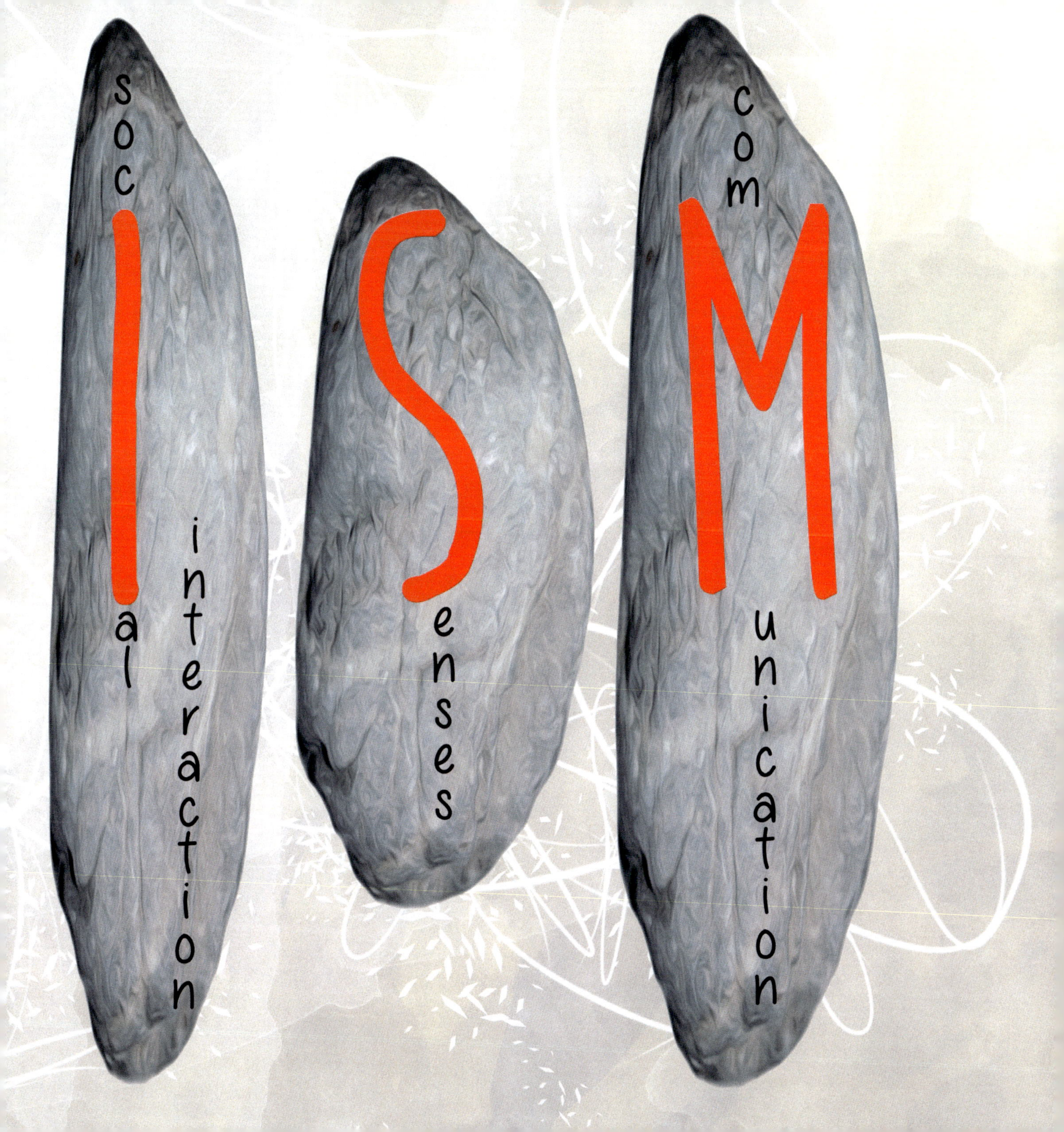

socIal
interaction
Senses
comMunication

"Autism?"

the little girl said, "I've never heard of it before. Will it grow me into an autumn tree that's always in a tizzy fit?"

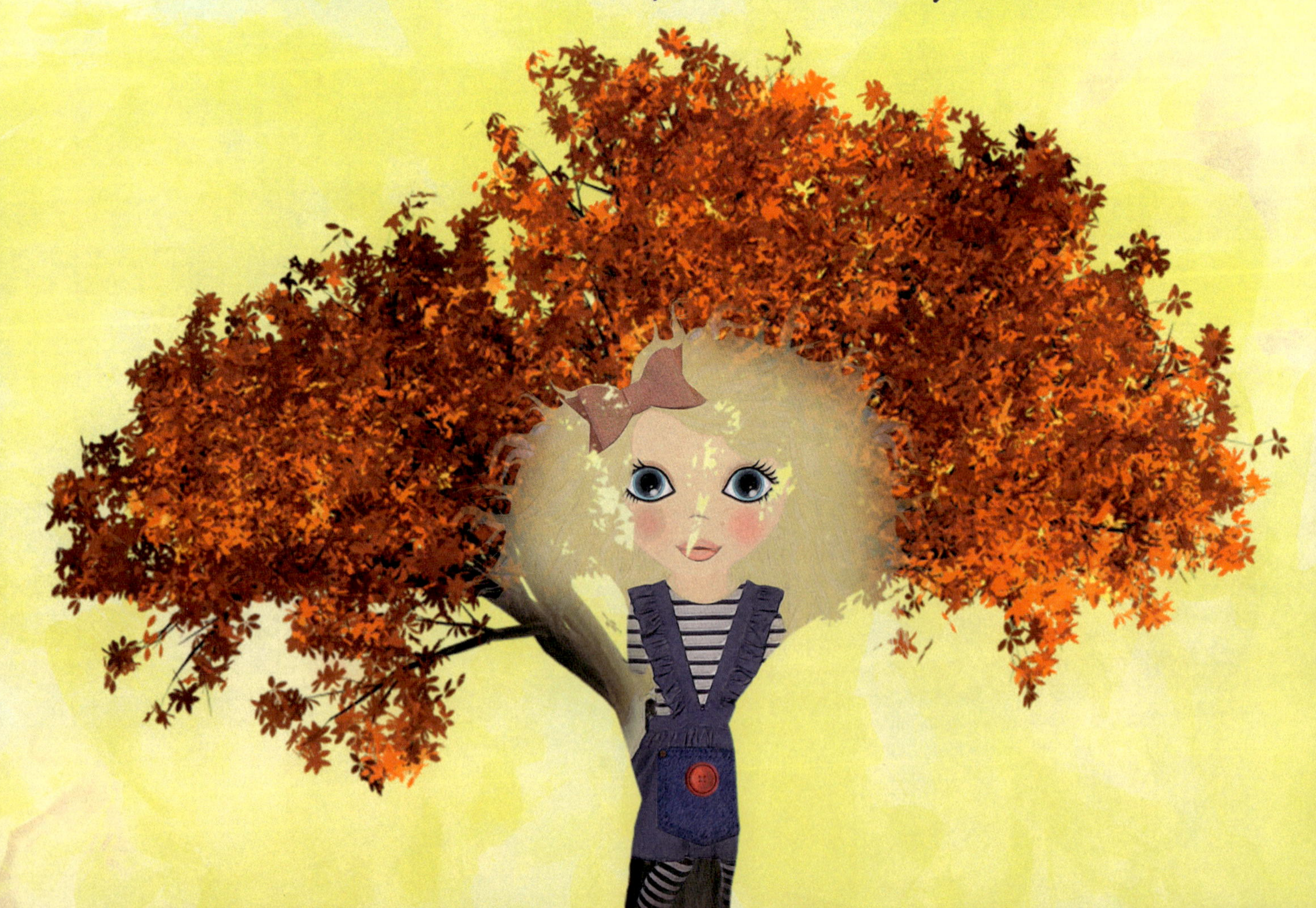

Mum reassured her, "It's perfectly ok to have autism. It's not something to be ashamed of. Lots of other children and grown-ups have it. Don't worry, it isn't a disease, or something you can die from and it definitely won't turn you into an autumn tree.

It simply means your brain was designed to work in a different way. Autism affects the way you experience the world and how you communicate and interact with others.

All autistic people share certain difficulties but being autistic affects everyone differently.

All these pebbles have different words on them: things that you have struggled with because of your autism, but, you must also know,

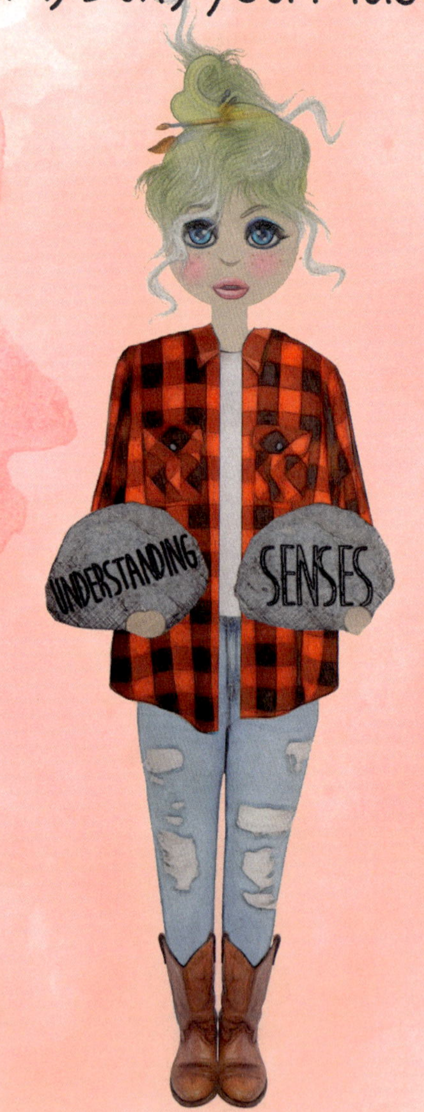

that just like these pebbles, autism has two sides."

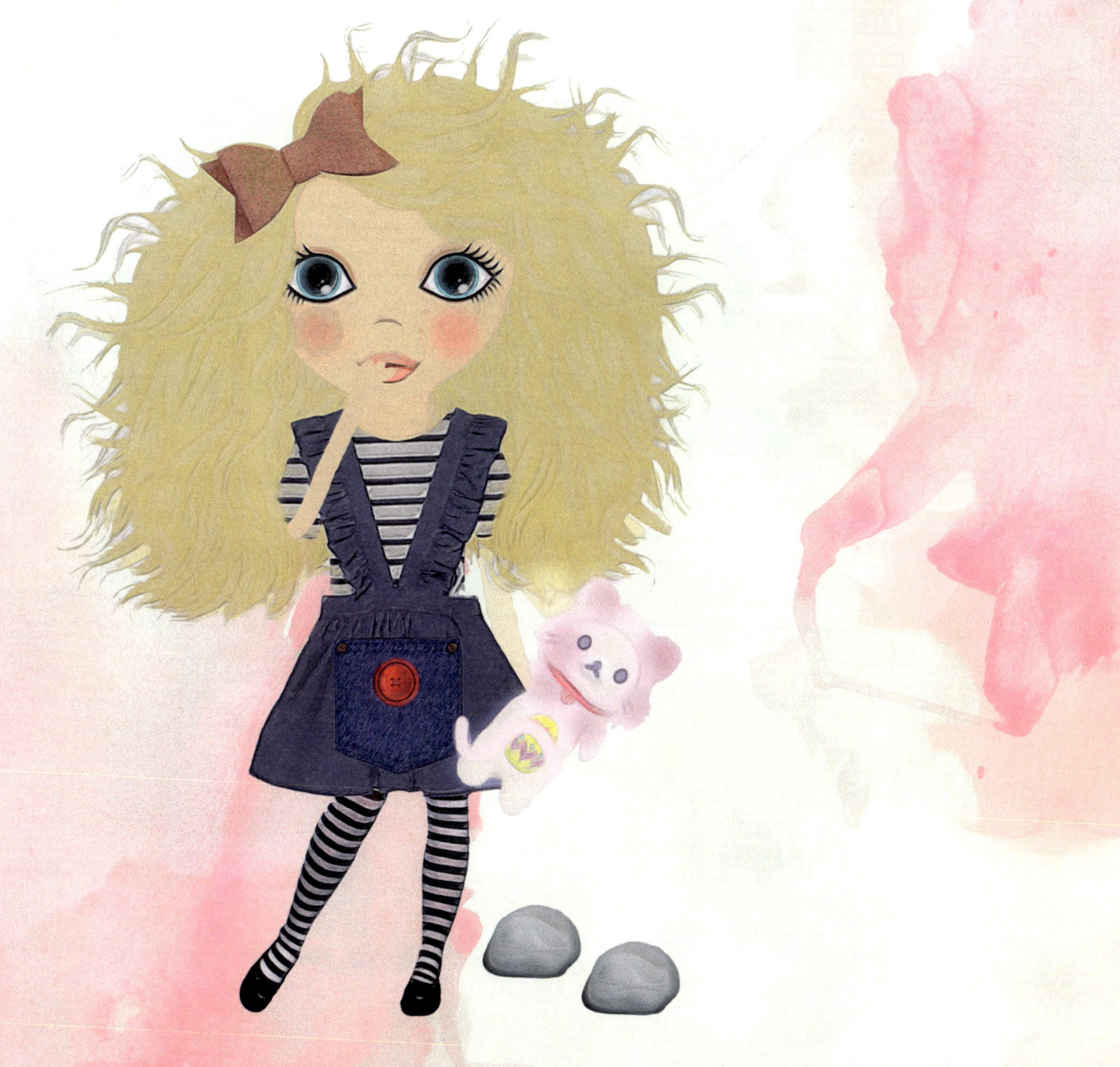

The little girl looked intrigued as Mum asked her to pick up a pebble.

She pointed to the pebble that said

understanding.

Mum lifted it and said,

"People with autism can find it difficult to understand what a bored or frowny face means or how people use their bodies to show how they feel.

This means it can be tough to interact appropriately in the classroom."

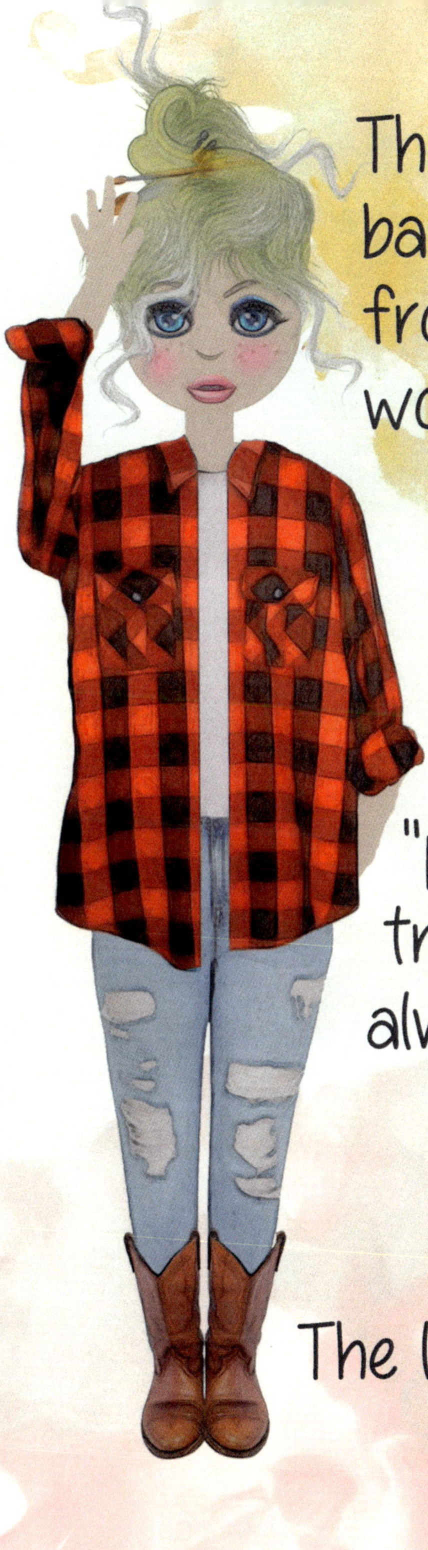

The little girl reached to see what the back said, just as Mum pulled a pencil from her hair and began to scratch words on the other side. She wrote,

trustworthy + loyal

and showed it to the little girl.

"Did you know," Mum explained, "people with autism are usually very trustworthy and loyal? In school you always return pencils you've borrowed and stand up for your classmates when someone is being mean."

The little girl smiled, took the pebble, and placed it on the ground.

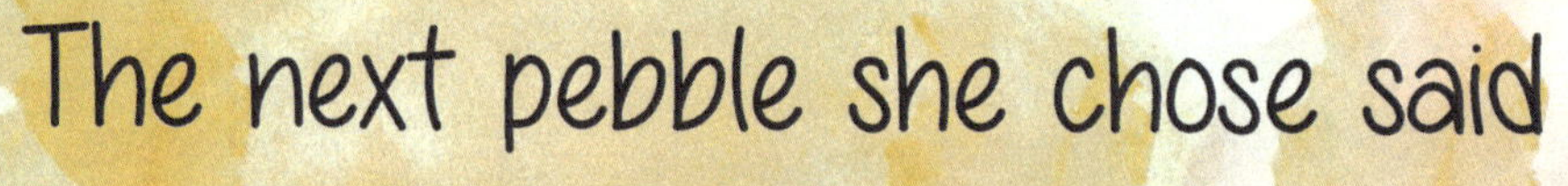

The next pebble she chose said

senses.

Mum smiled and gave the pebble a hug:

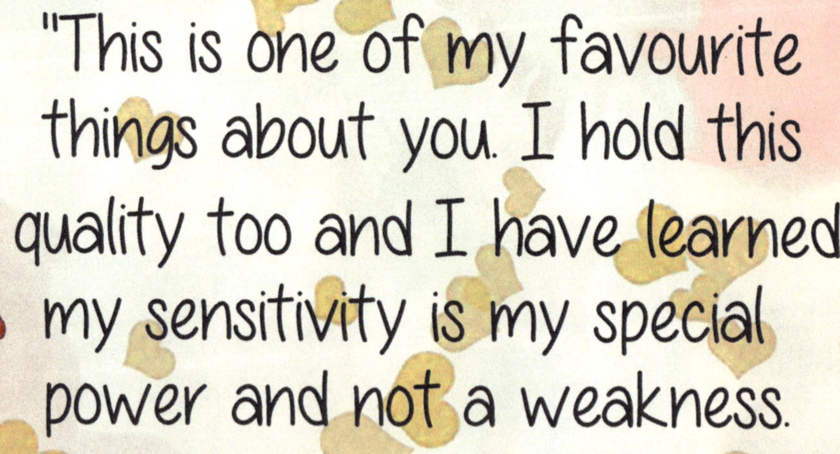

"This is one of my favourite things about you. I hold this quality too and I have learned my sensitivity is my special power and not a weakness.

Sometimes we experience difficult emotions more intensely than others, and we must learn to protect ourselves, but there is always a flip side - two sides - just like this pebble.

The flip side is: we get to feel all the good emotions more deeply.

This is what makes us creative; by accepting and focusing our sensitivity we can bring beautiful changes into the world that others might not see."

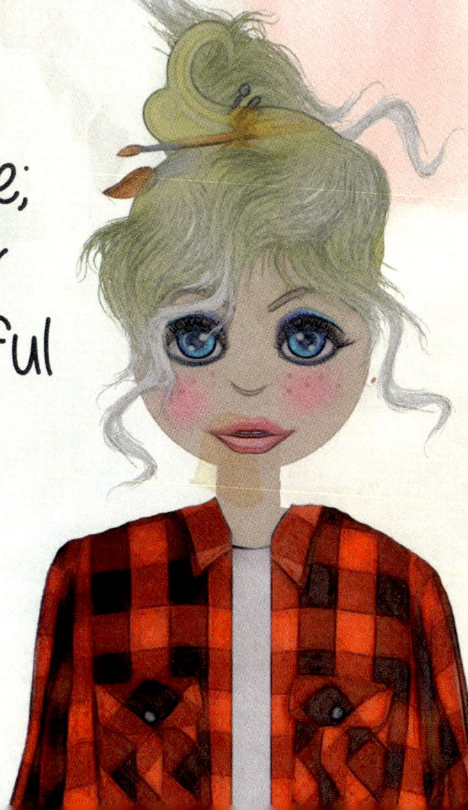

Mum took the pebble and scratched
creative.
"I love how sensitive, gentle and empathetic you are with little kids you meet. The imaginative games you play make them feel instantly at ease. So, you see, you're already using your sensitivity to bring good to other people.

Did you know, thousands of years ago people who were very sensitive, just like you, were highly respected? They could see, taste, smell and sense things other people couldn't. They understood nature in an amazing way, so sensed storms and warned people to take shelter from the crashing lightning and threatening rain. Their senses made them survivors."

The little girl felt proud, took the pebble, and placed it beside the others.

She lifted the next pebble and handed it to her mum. It said

change.

"You know how you sometimes find change difficult, like the time Grandma bought you a new pussycat and you didn't want to play with it? Well, the other side of the pebble should say **reliable.** When you grow up and have a job you'll be brilliant when there are repetitive things to do because you're passionate and like everything to be organized and perfect."

Mum lifted another pebble that said

repetitive patterns,

wrote **passionate** on the back, and set it amongst the other pebbles.

The little girl asked about the pebble that said

communication.

"Oh," said Mum, "the other side of communication is your fantastic ability to tell me lots of details from memory, like the names of your toys." Mum flipped the pebble over, wrote **memory** and placed it with the others. Mum and the little girl wrote on the other sides of a few more pebbles until they came to the last one. It said:

social interaction.

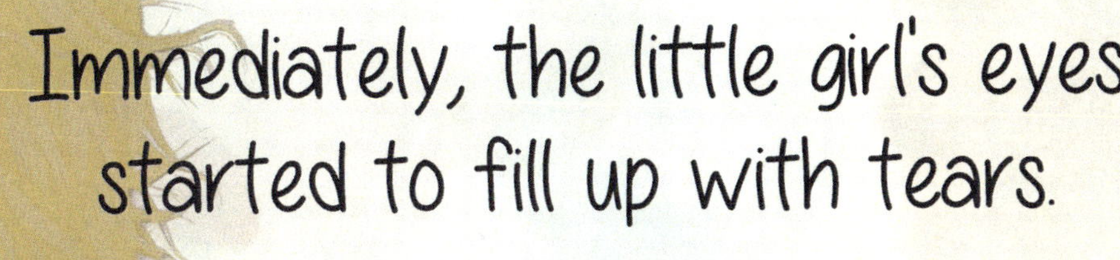

Immediately, the little girl's eyes started to fill up with tears.

"This means I can't make friends very well, doesn't it?" she asked sadly.

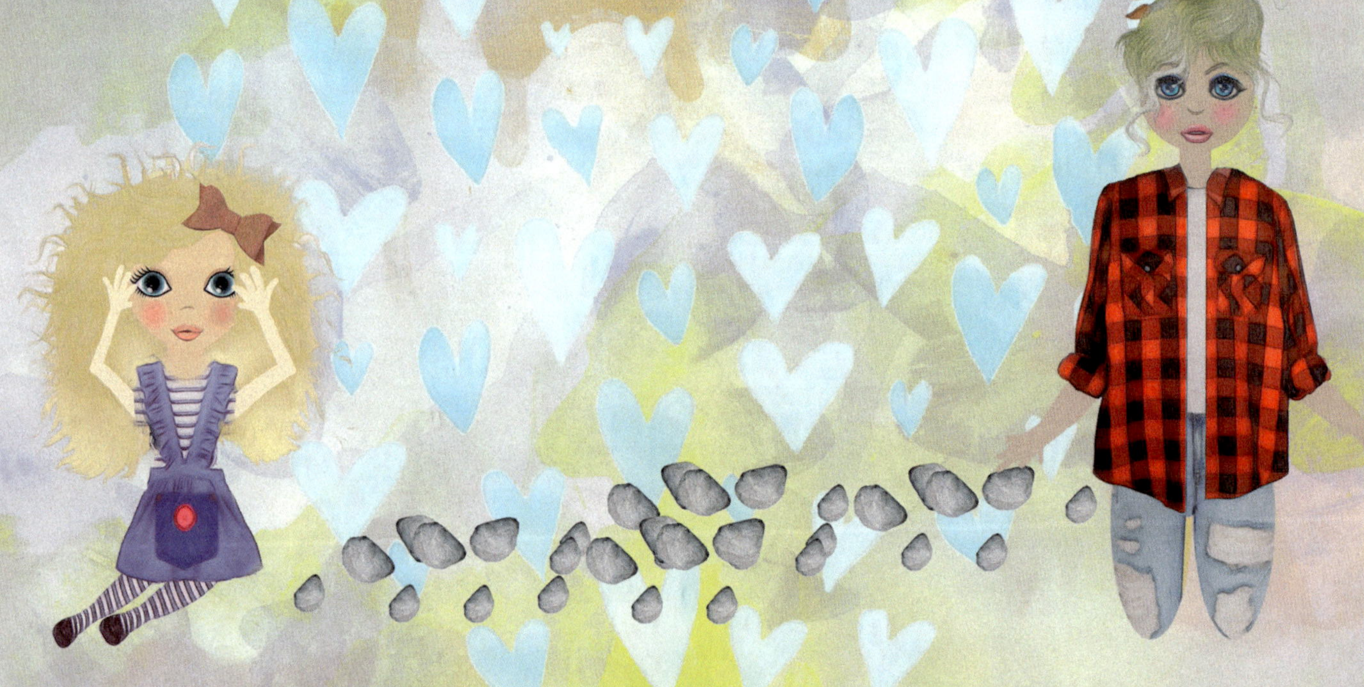

They looked at the pebble together and Mum started, "It can mean that, but it has another side to it that's good."

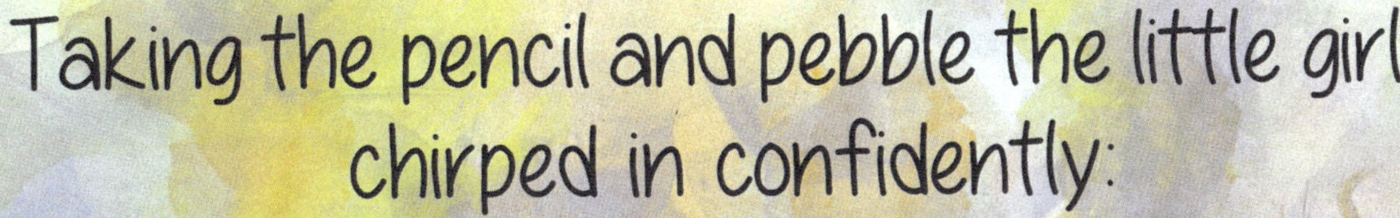

Taking the pencil and pebble the little girl chirped in confidently:

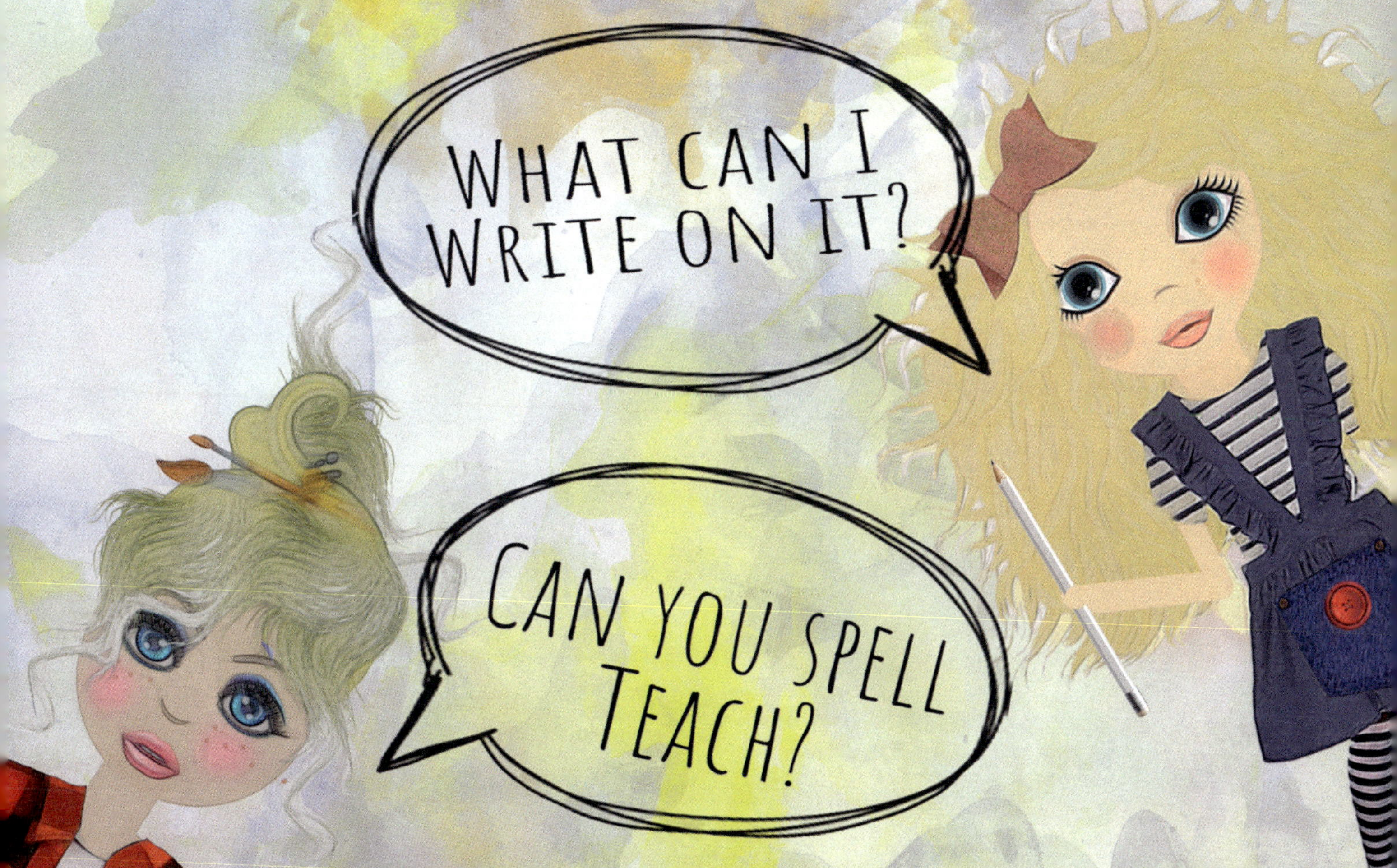

WHAT CAN I WRITE ON IT?

CAN YOU SPELL TEACH?

The little girl nodded and scratched **teach** onto the pebble. She looked at Mum and waited patiently to hear what she had to say.

"You have the ability to teach others to live as they are and not pretend to be someone they are not. You can teach others that fitting in isn't important; just be yourself. What matters is what you love and are passionate about.

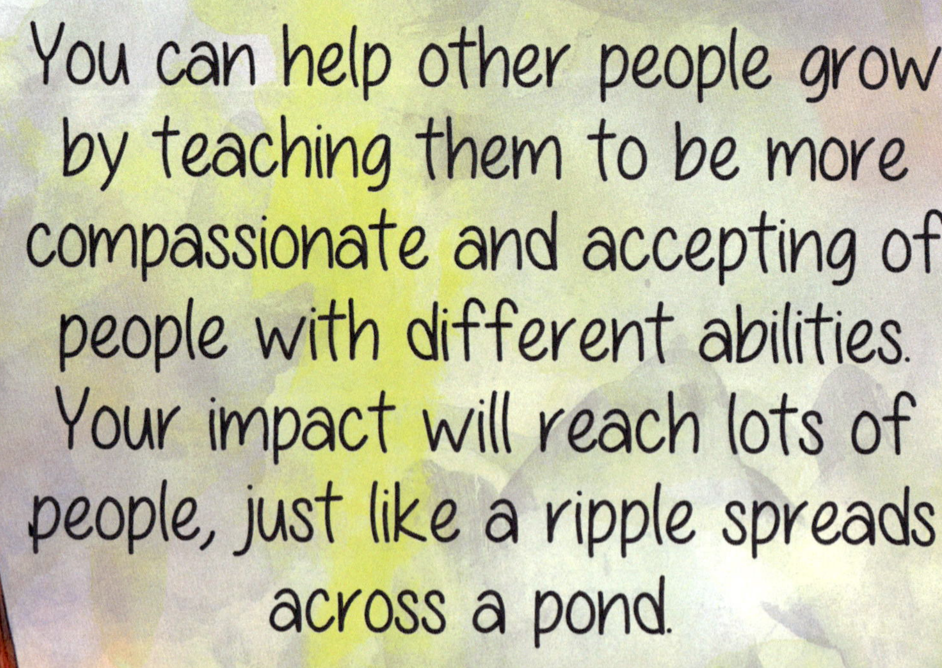

You can help other people grow by teaching them to be more compassionate and accepting of people with different abilities. Your impact will reach lots of people, just like a ripple spreads across a pond.

What you have taught me are lessons I wouldn't have found in a book. Being your mum has released me from a lifetime of 'should' and offered me a new world called 'is', and I love every bit of it - no more expectations - instead, treasuring your uniqueness."

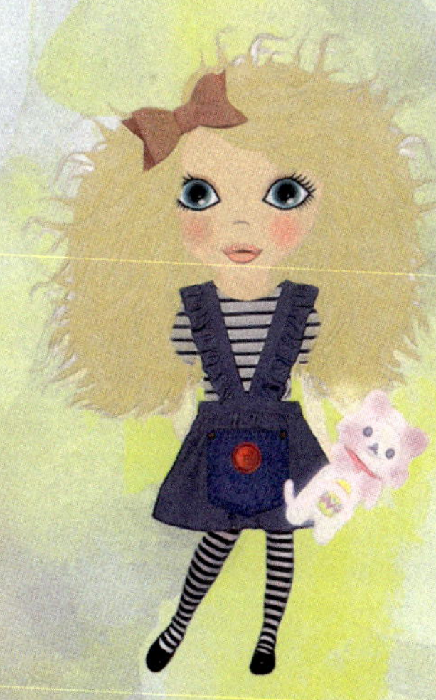

The little girl gave her mum a hug and set the pebble with the others.

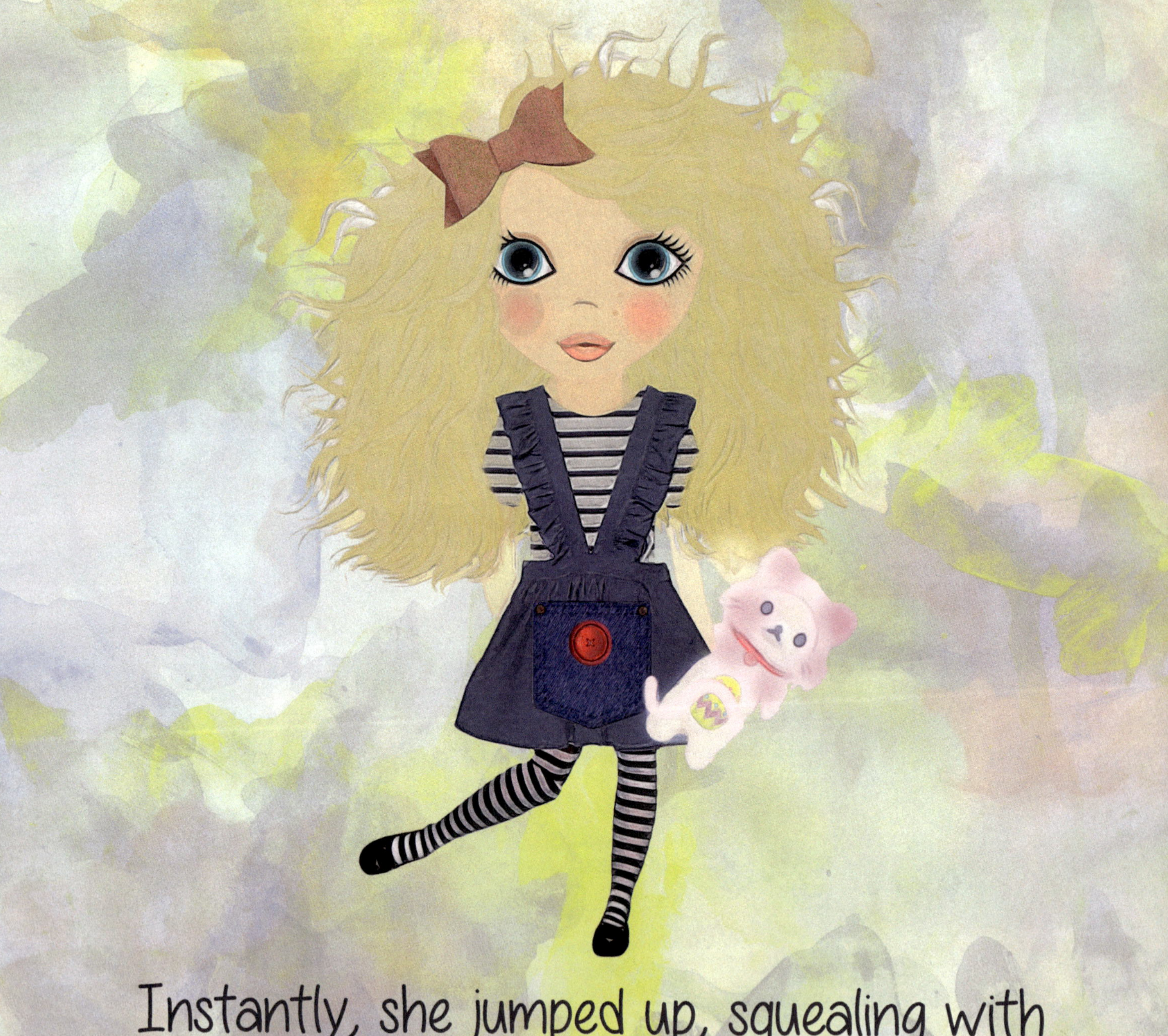

Instantly, she jumped up, squealing with excitement, "Mummy! The pebbles are spelling out another word!"

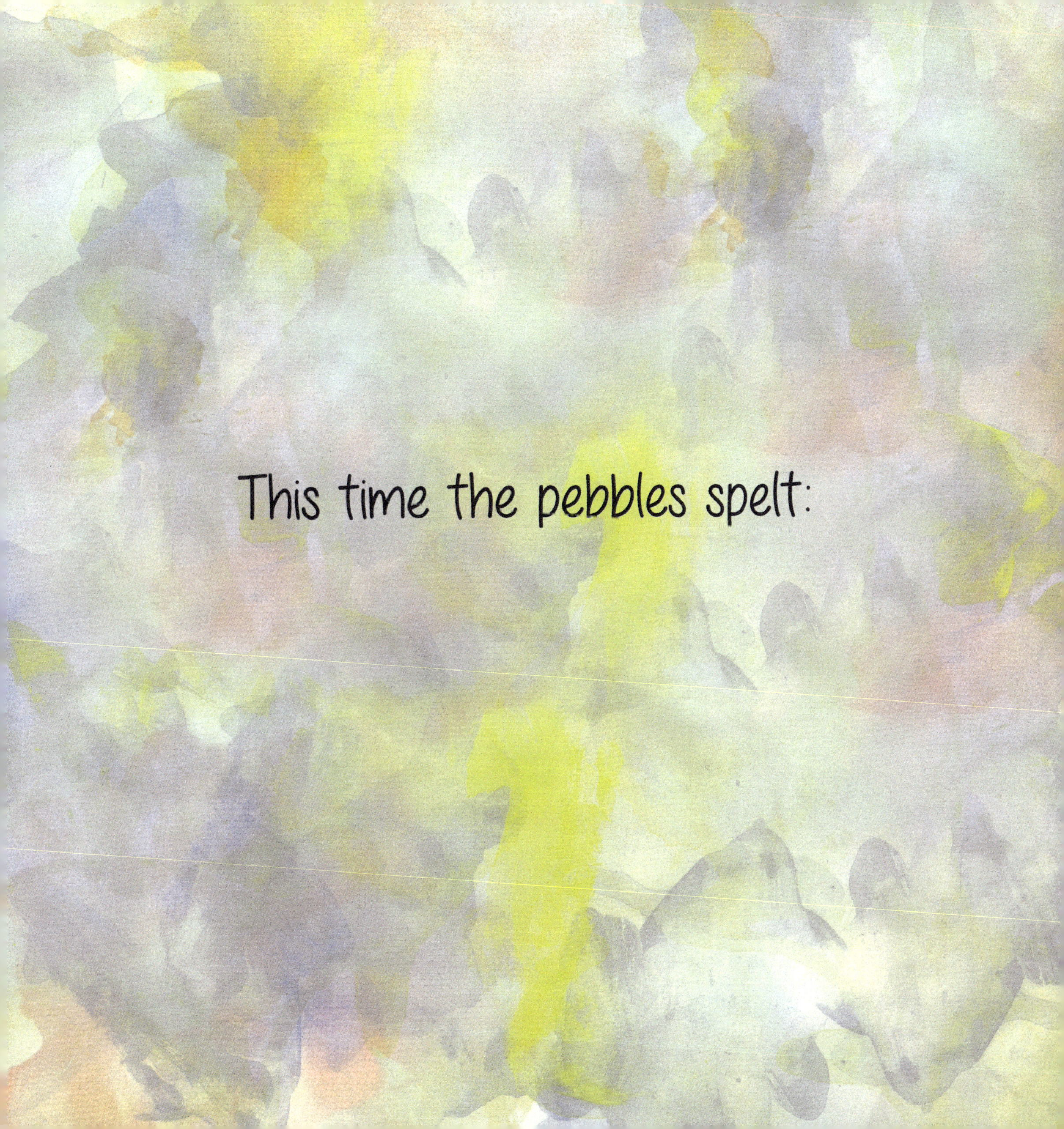

This time the pebbles spelt:

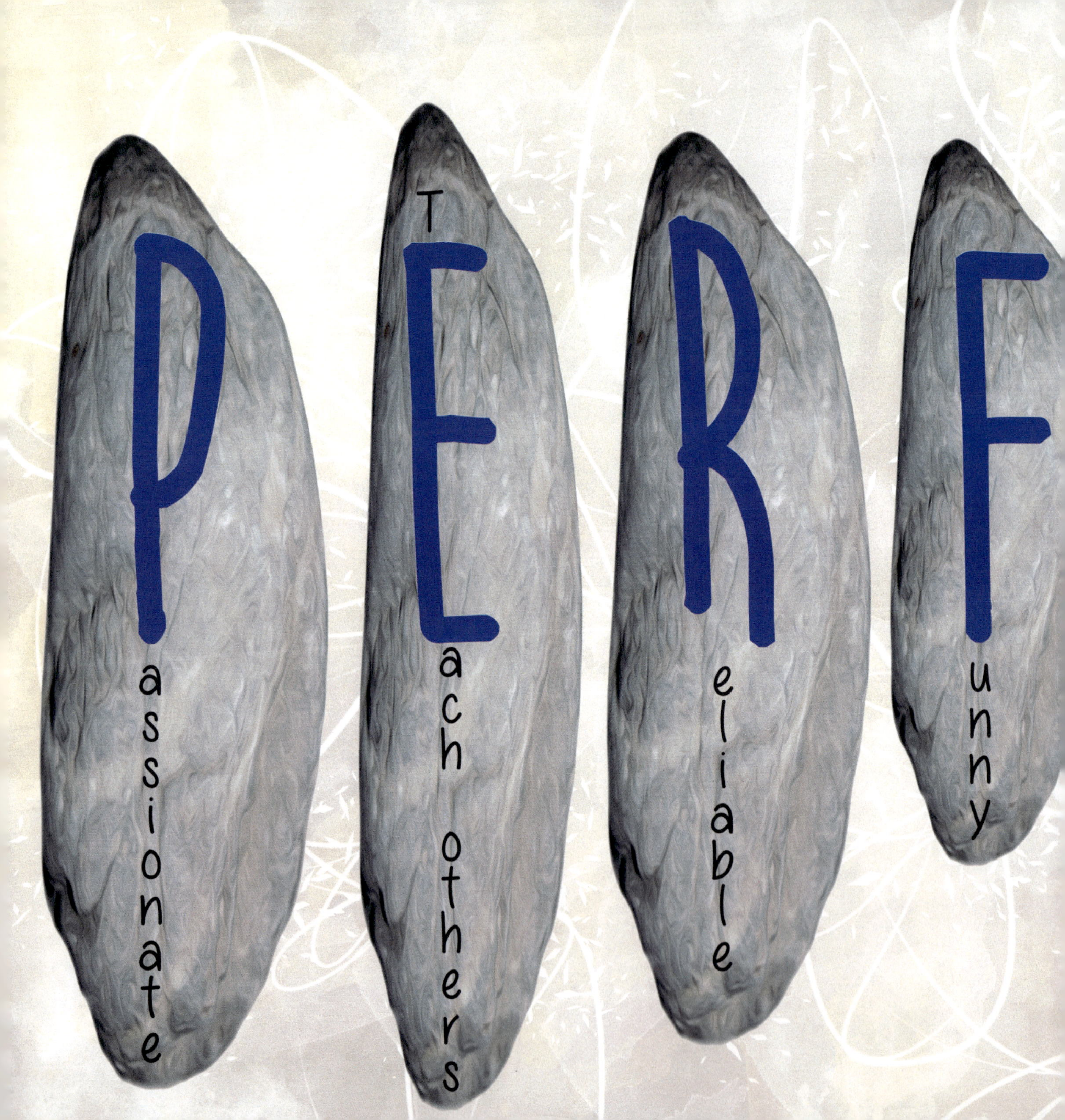
Passionate
Teach others
Reliable
Funny

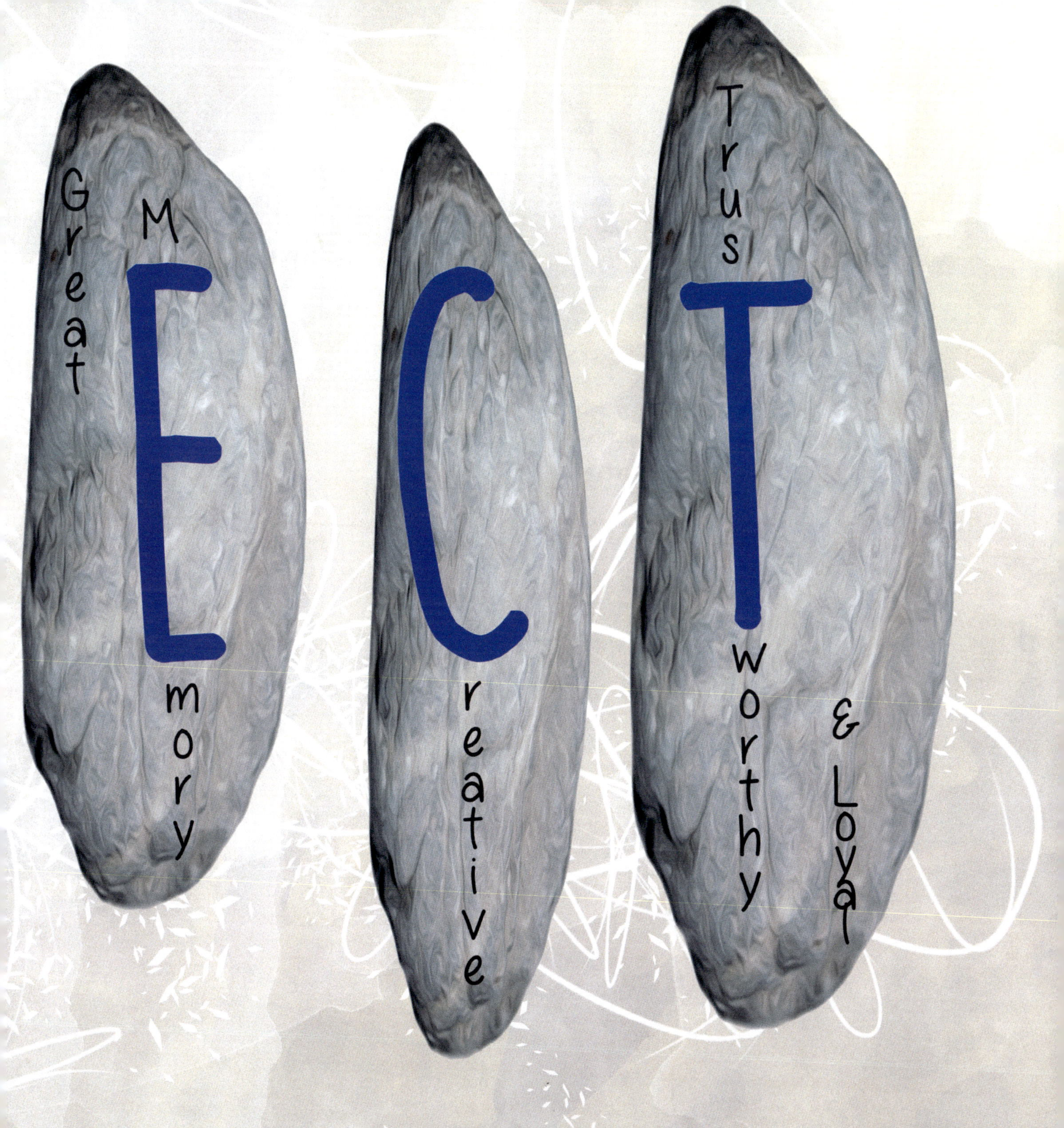
Great
Memory
E
C
Creative
Trus
T
Tworthy
& Loyal

Mum and the little girl hugged each other tightly while Mum whispered in her ear: "Now you know your secret, it's up to you if you want to tell others. Just remember, when you think things are tough, on the other side there are so many positives, just like there are two sides to every pebble.

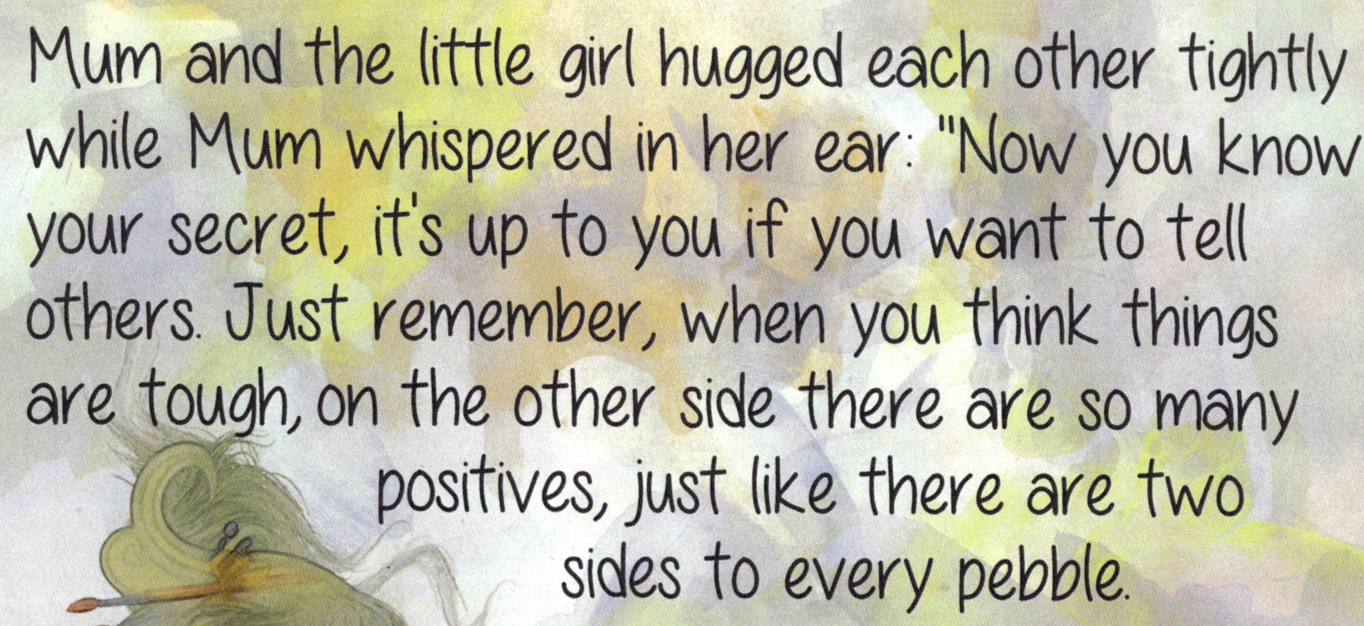

YOU are PERFECT.

Don't ever forget."

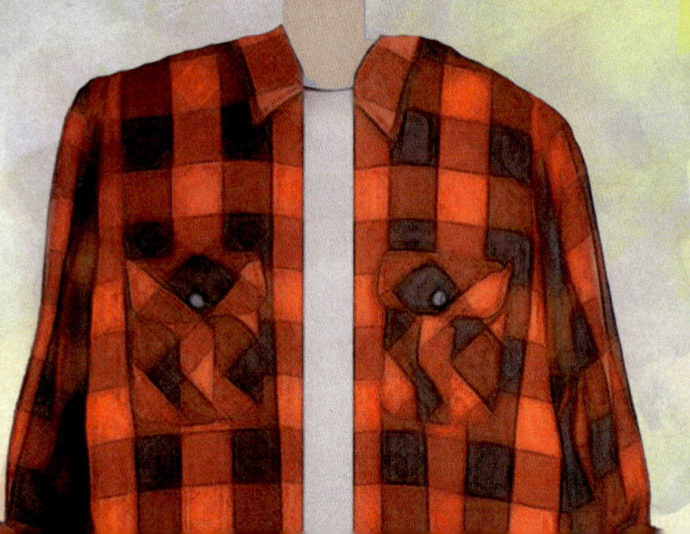

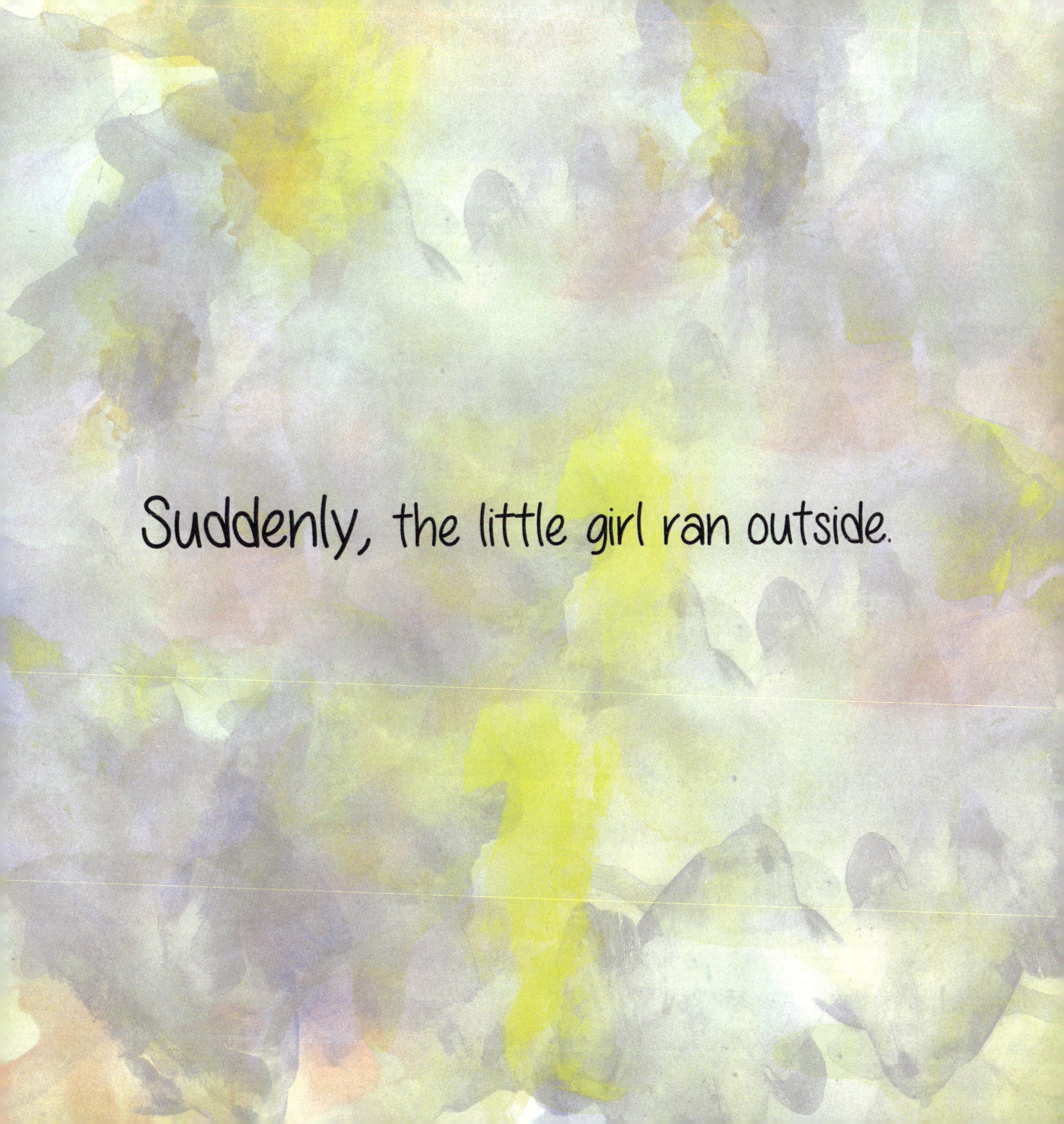

Suddenly, the little girl ran outside.

She came back with a wild poppy flower, handed it to her mummy and said,

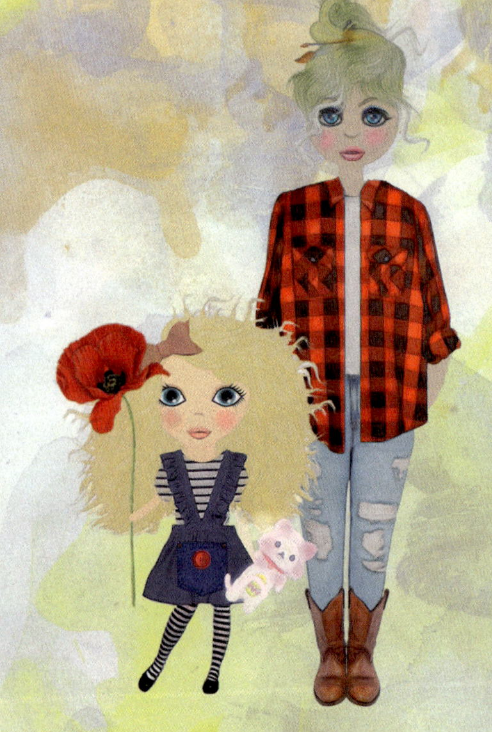

"You are the best mummy I've ever had; if I could pick a cloud I would give it to you.

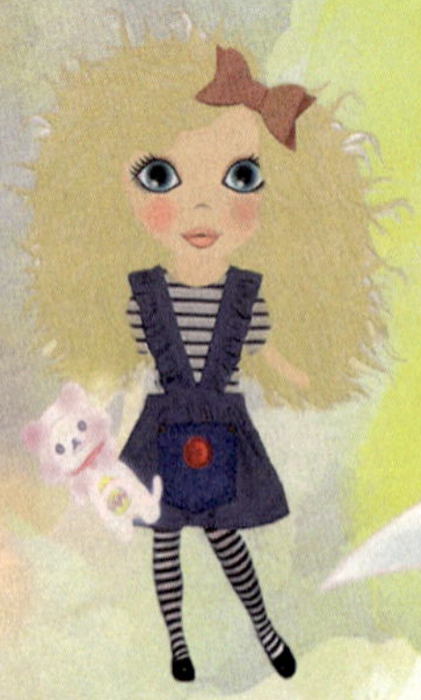

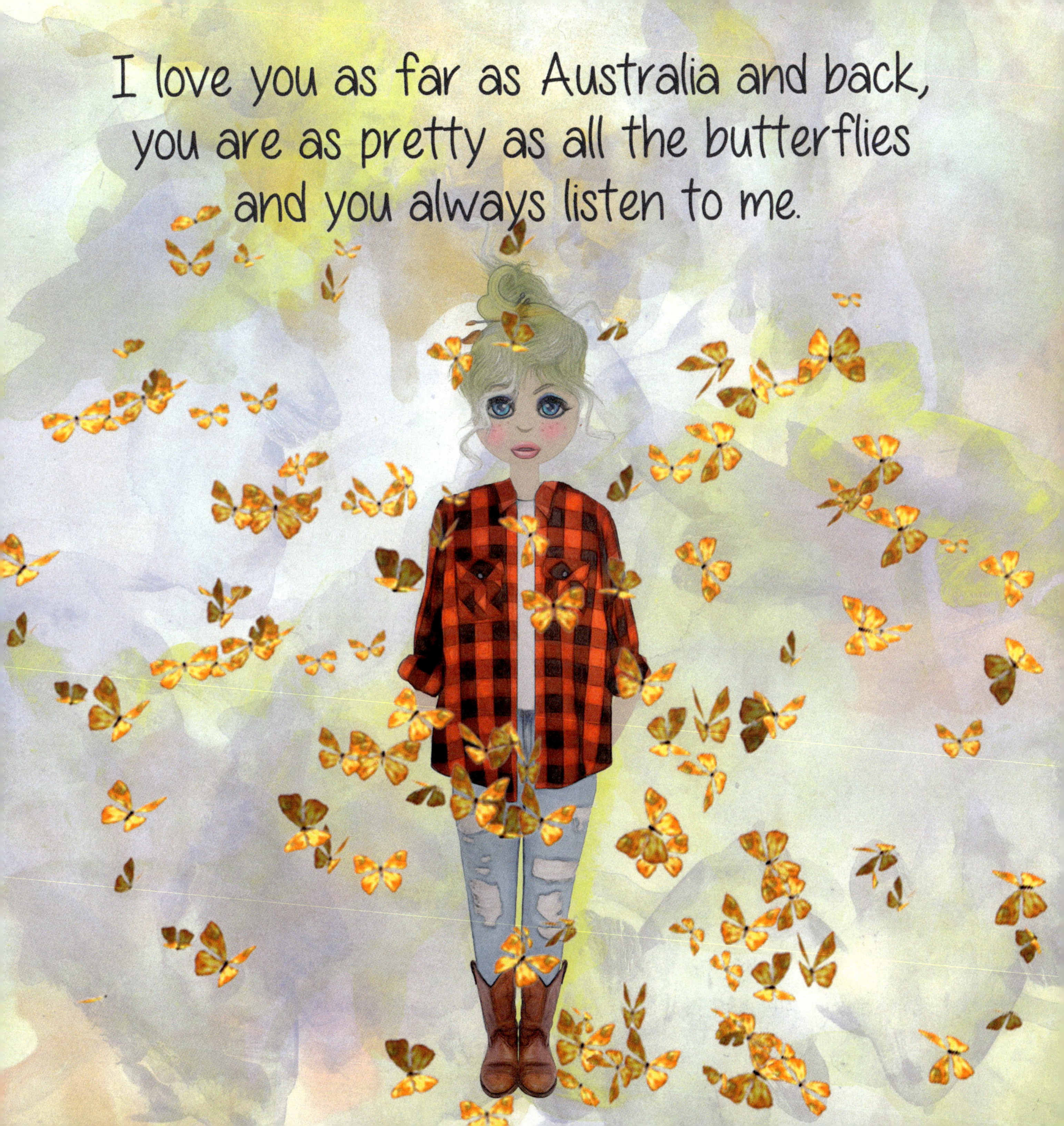

I love you as far as Australia and back,
you are as pretty as all the butterflies
and you always listen to me.

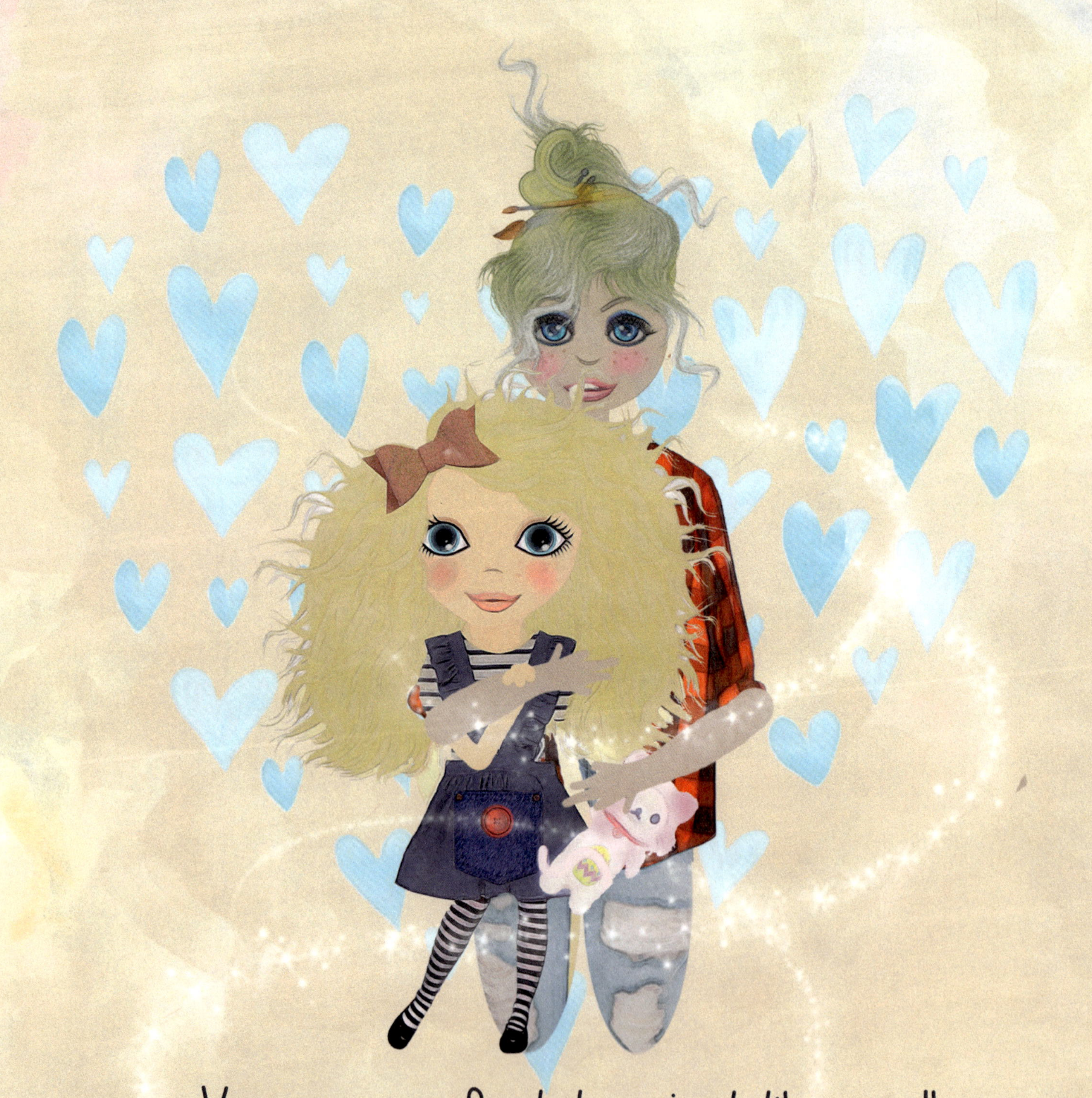

You are perfect too, just like me."

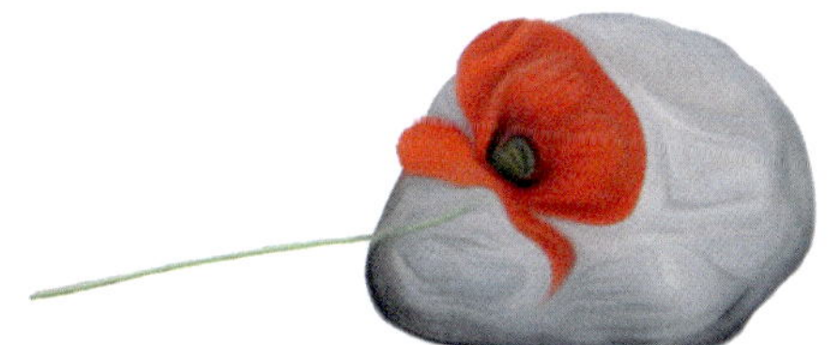

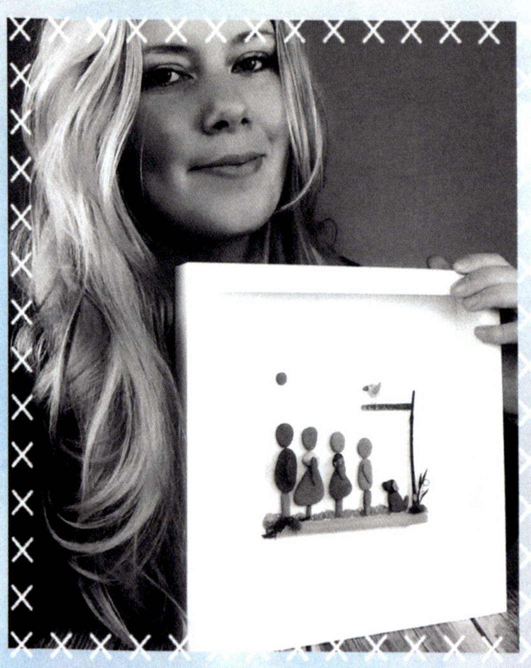

Author's note.

Award-winning and worldwide selling artist Anita Morrison (AMor Rustic Arts) has set down her paint brushes and dusted off her computer to create a captivating story to reveal compassionately, her daughter's autism diagnosis to her.

Her daughter was diagnosed with autism at age three, and everyday since Anita wondered how she was going to tell her daughter that she had autism.

Anita explains:

"Since visual aids are proven to be beneficial for autistic children, I looked at numerous other picture books for help, but the majority were too factual and quite frightening for kids. I wanted something that both introduced my daughter to autism and also empowered her."

It is Anita's hope that the mainstream education system gets appropriate funding and training to adapt to meet the autistic community's needs, so that schools will no longer have to push our autistic children to fit the standards of normality but instead, enhance their existing skills and talents, which will boost their mental wellbeing and self-confidence.

You can find out more about Anita's artwork by searching 'AMor Rustic Arts' on Facebook or by visiting her site www.amorrusticarts.com

To find out more about this book search 'The Pebble Secret' on Facebook or visit the website www.thepebblesecret.com

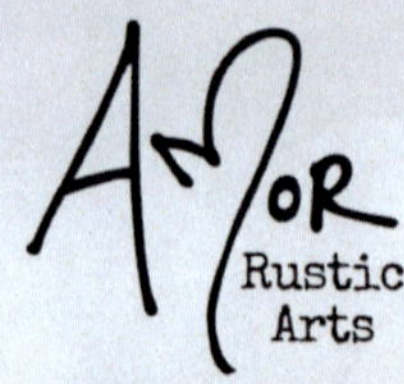

Made in the USA
Columbia, SC
28 March 2021

35212436R00040